Resident's Handbook of Medical Quality and Safety

Levi (Levan) Atanelov
Editor

Resident's Handbook of Medical Quality and Safety

Springer

Editor
Levi (Levan) Atanelov
Johns Hopkins Hospital
Baltimore, MD, USA

ISBN 978-3-319-24188-3 ISBN 978-3-319-24190-6 (eBook)
DOI 10.1007/978-3-319-24190-6

Library of Congress Control Number: 2015960364

Printed on acid-free paper

This Springer imprint is published by Springer Nature
The registered company is Springer International Publishing AG Switzerland

To Dassi, a muse
of inspiration and
a bedrock of support.
To Deda and Babo,
humbling paragons
of human potential.

Introduction/Preface: How to Use This Book

Who is this book for: **residency program directors, medical residents, attending physicians, nurses, physical and occupational therapists, and other clinicians, as well as trainees interested in pursuing these career paths.**

What is medical safety and quality improvement? Per Dr. Pronovost: "The goal of quality and safety interventions is to partner with patients their loved ones and others to (1) eliminate harm, (2) continuously improve patient outcomes and experience, (3) eliminate waste; as such, we group our work into three areas: (1) safety; (2) performance on externally reported measures and outcomes; and (3) value. The tools we use are multiple including lean, informatics, human factors etc...."

Scope of the book: this is a small pocketbook intended to help promote the engagement of current and future clinicians (e.g., program directors, nurses, residents, attending physicians, physical and occupational therapists, etc....) in safety and medical quality initiatives. We will not demonstrate the relevance of medical safety and quality improvement or its current impact on healthcare. **The overall philosophy of the book is to present the information in a condensed, get-out-and-do-it-now format for busy clinicians who want to jump-start a project.** We are featuring some of the tools often employed in medical safety and quality improvement (QI) studies as well as some sample medical quality and safety projects undertaken by clinicians at Johns Hopkins Hospital and the Armstrong Institute of Patient Safety and Quality. **Please note, this book is not meant to teach everything you need to know about implementing QI work, but is meant to**

be a springboard, such that once some fundamental concepts have been clarified, you can look online or seek out professionals with more expertise in the field. Also note that even though this book provides an introduction on technical aspects of Lean Six Sigma and statistics, it is very likely that additional help may be required. In order to promote the field of medical safety and quality improvement, help foster collaboration between clinicians engaged in QI projects, give further assistance to the readers of this handbook, and provide clarification of the material covered in the book as well as additional support for specific QI interventions, we have created an online forum medicalqualityandsafetyforum.com. The forum is an opportunity for beginners in QI to seek guidance and for more seasoned QI professionals to develop mentorship relationships and share their knowledge (advanced QI practitioners will benefit from increased name recognition in the cyberspace in reward for their assistance).

What is in this book? Sample projects in the book are designed to demonstrate the roadblocks and successes, as well as methodology and tools commonly employed in safety and quality endeavors. **We try to emphasize the process rather than the outcome in presenting the sample projects. Attending level projects can help differentiate between resident and attending level of work and develop realistic expectations.** Chapters on how to scope a project can further assist with goal-setting. There are two such chapters as poorly scoped projects are a common downfall of many QI initiatives. The book also provides a short introduction to the field of medical quality improvement and an overview of common QI tools, responsible consumption of evidence-based medicine in academic publications, team and project management, communication tools, as well as more technical aspects of QI initiatives (e.g., statistics and statistical software). Overall efforts were made to balance between the topics covering "people skills" to engage and maintain quality interventions and the technical skills to demonstrate in a data-driven manner the effect of the interventions. Again, these chapters will not substitute the services of a trained statistician, project manager, or clinical scientist. A short introduction to the statistical language R can be helpful for running basic statistical calculations (this is the most robust statistical language that is *free*, to the best of my knowledge). Since much of QI involves assessment of subjective human experiences and culture of the healthcare system, a small chapter on writing surveys is attached. Please note that this is not THE QI TEXTBOOK, but a pocketbook to supplement formal training by other means.

Administrative perspectives on clinician participation in QI interventions can help residency program directors and hospital administrators frame the utility of medical safety and quality improvement in their institutions as well as learn about some of the models utilized here at Johns Hopkins. **I am infinitely grateful to Dr. Redonda Miller and Dr. R.S. Mayer for their contribution toward these goals.**

Why am I interested in safety and quality improvement? Prior to medical training I studied in Israel Talmudic principles of Jewish Medical Ethics (JME), *Mussar* (a systematized approach for continual self-improvement) and concepts of *Tikkun HaOlam* (improving the world). From intellectual/ethical perspective, *do no wrong* and *beneficence* mean that every physician is responsible to provide safe ("do no wrong") and high-quality (beneficence) medical care. Simply put, we all intuitively agree that automotive mechanics should take responsibility for providing quality work on car breaks they service. If so, what does that mean for clinicians engaged in care of human beings? From heart/personal perspective (and this is why many of us choose careers in medicine), I, like many of my colleague clinicians, have been privy to the unfortunate consequences of healthcare failures and would like to do whatever is in my power to prevent their future reoccurrence. We all dream of changing the world; perhaps this handbook can motivate positive changes in the world of medicine and the patients we serve.

Debt of Gratitude: **I am forever grateful to my teacher and source of inspiration, Dr. Peter Pronovost, for creating the Armstrong Institute of Patient Safety and Quality, developing a Fellowship in Patient Safety and Quality Improvement, teaching us about this exciting field, and for encouraging and assisting me with creating this book.** Similarly, I owe a debt of gratitude to Dr. Paul Nagy for running the Fellowship of Medical Safety and Quality Improvement at Hopkins and for many instructors who came and spoke with us during the fellowship training. Last but not least, my thanks go out to Dr. Hoyer, my friend and mentor in QI.

Baltimore, MD, USA Levi (Levan) Atanelov

Contents

Part I: Background to Medical Quality Improvement and Safety

1 **Basic Quality Improvement Terminology** 3
Levi (Levan) Atanelov

2 **History of QI and Safety in the USA** 9
Sina Parizadeh

3 **Safety Risk Management Principles from the Federal Aviation Administration** 17
Benyamin Wise

4 **Human Factors Engineering for Quality Improvement and Research in Health Care** 21
Ayse P. Gurses

5 **The Role of Informatics and Electronic Health Record in Current Medical Practice: What Are the Benefits of Medical Informatics to the Clinician?** 29
Andre Cassell

Part II: Perspectives for Residency Program Directors and Hospital Administration

6 **The Importance of Resident Involvement in Quality Improvement: An Investment in Our Future** 35
Redonda G. Miller

7 **Residency Program Director's Perspective on Patient Safety and Quality Improvement** 39
R. Samuel Mayer

8 House Staff Patient Safety Quality Council 49
Michelle Sharp

Part III: Sample QI Projects

9 Promoting Early Mobility for Hospitalized Patients: A Quality Improvement (QI) Project 55
Levi (Levan) Atanelov and Erik Hoyer

10 Heart Sounds: Use of Audio Recordings to Improve Patient Discharge Communication 67
Stacey L. Schott

11 Smoking Cessation in Pregnancy and Beyond: A Quality Improvement (QI) Project 81
Marielle S. Gross

12 Facilitating Early-In-Day Discharge for Multiple Sclerosis Patients Treated with Intravenous Methylprednisolone: A Quality Improvement (QI) Project 89
John C. Probasco

13 Improving Compliance with Vaccination Core Measures 99
Susan Peterson and Brent Petty

14 Implementing Early Rehabilitation in the ICU to Improve Patient Outcomes 109
Ibtehal Kimawi and Dale M. Needham

15 Developing a Consistent Multidisciplinary Delivery of Therapy Care System for Acute Care Therapy Services 115
Julie Kreif

16 Quality Improvement and CAUTI Project: A Nursing Approach 127
Amber Renaud

17 Streamlining the Stat Medication Process: An Interdisciplinary Quality Improvement Project 131
Melinda D. Sawyer, Jennifer V. Gillespie, Denice L. Duda, and Robert E. Hody

Part IV: Consuming and Producing Academic Literature

18 Publishing Your Work: A Bird's-Eye View Outline 145
Levi (Levan) Atanelov

19 Tips for Effective Literature Searching 151
Carrie Price

20 Resources for Grading the Evidence, Appraisal, Writing, and Publishing 163
Carrie Price

21 Basic Principles of Consuming Academic Literature 169
Zaza Atanelov

Part V: Implementing Quality Improvement Interventions

22 Generating Creative Ideas as a Group for Quality Improvement 185
Sharon H. Kim

23 Scope 193
Kevin C. Platt

24 How to Select and Scope a Project 201
Laura Winner and Richard Hill

25 Communication Tools in Healthcare: Basics 217
Solomon Rojhani and R. Samuel Mayer

26 Project Management: Basics 231
Solomon Rojhani

27 Team Management in Healthcare: Basics 253
Solomon Rojhani

28 Quality Improvement Tools: A Potpourri 263
Charles A. Odonkor

29 Quality Improvement (QI): Implementing QI Tools 275
Charles A. Odonkor

30 Lean Sigma Case Study 299
Richard Hill

Part VI: Technical Aspects of Quality Improvement

31 QI Tools: Epidemiology Basics – Application of Epidemiological Tools to Patient Safety and Quality 329
Ruchika Goel and Raminder Chadha

32 Introduction to Data Analysis for QI Projects 339
Marlis Gonzalez-Fernandez

33 Survey Methodology 351
Phillip H. Phan

34 Using R for Statistics: A Beginner's Manual 361
Andre Cassell

Erratum E1

Index 389

Contributors

Levi (Levan) Atanelov, MD, MS Department of Physical Medicine and Rehabilitation, Johns Hopkins Hospital, Baltimore, MA, USA

Zaza Atanelov, BA School of Medicine, School of Health Sciences and Practice, New York Medical College, Vahalla, NY, USA

Andre Cassell, MD Department of Physical Medicine and Rehabilitation, John Hopkins Hospital, Baltimore, MD, USA

Raminder Chadha, PharmD Johns Hopkins Hospital, Baltimore, MD

Denice L. Duda, BSN, MHA, RPHQ Department of Quality Improvement, The John Hopkins Hospital, Baltimore, MD, USA

Jennifer V. Gillespie, PharmD Department of Pharmacy, The Johns Hopkins Hospital, Baltimore, MD, USA

Ruchika Goel, MD Division of Pediatric Hematology, The Johns Hopkins Hospital, Baltimore, MD, USA

Marlis Gonzalez-Fernandez, MD, PhD Department of Physical Medicine and Rehabilitation, John Hopkins Hospital, Baltimore, MD, USA

Marielle S. Gross, MD Department of Gynecology and Obstetrics, John Hopkins University School of Medicine, Baltimore, MD, USA

Ayse P. Gurses, PhD Hopkins Bloomberg School of Public Health, Baltimore, MD, USA

Department of Anesthesiology and Critical Medicine, Johns Hopkins Hospital, Baltimore, MD, USA

Richard Hill, BS Armstrong Institute for Patient Safety and Quality, John Hopkins Hospital, Baltimore, MD, USA

Robert E. Hody, MS, CMBB Armstrong Institute for Patient Safety and Quality, John Hopkins University School of Medicine, Baltimore, MD, USA

Erik Hoyer, MD Department of Physical Medicine and Rehabilitation, John Hopkins Hospital, Baltimore, MD, USA

Sharon H. Kim, PhD Carey Business School and Armstrong Institute for Patient Safety and Quality, John Hopkins Hospital, Baltimore, MD, USA

Ibtehal Kimawi, MBBS Department of Pulmonary and Critical Care Medicine, John Hopkins University School of Medicine, Baltimore, MD, USA

Julie Kreif, PT, MBA Department of Physical Medicine and Rehabilitation, The John Hopkins Hospital, Baltimore, MD, USA

R. Samuel Mayer, MD Department of Physical Medicine and Rehabilitation, John Hopkins University School of Medicine, Baltimore, MD, USA

Redonda G. Miller, MD, MBA Department of Medical Affairs, The John Hopkins Hospital, Balitmore, MD, USA

Dale M. Needham, FCPA, MD, PhD Department of Pulmonary and Critical Care Medicine, John Hopkins University School of Medicine, Baltimore, MD, USA

Charles A. Odonkor, MD, MA Department of Physical Medicine and Rehabilitation, Johns Hopkins Hospital, Baltimore, MD, USA

Sina Parizadeh, PhD Ner Israel Rabbinical College, Baltimore, MD, USA

Susan Peterson, MD Department of Emergency Medicine, John Hopkins University School of Medicine, Baltimore, MD, USA

Brent Petty, MD Department of Medicine, John Hopkins Hospital, Baltimore, MD, USA

Phillip H. Phan, PhD Carey Business School, John Hopkins Hospital, Baltimore, MD, USA

Kevin C. Platt, PT, DPT, MBA, FACHE Department of Impatient Rehabilitation, MedStar Good Samaritan Hospital, Baltimore, MD, USA

Carrie Price, MLS Welch Medical Library, Johns Hopkins University, School of Medicine, Baltimore, MD, USA

John C. Probasco, MD Department of Neurology, John Hopkins Hospital, Baltimore, MD, USA

Amber Renaud, AS, RN, BSN Department of Rehabilitation, MedStar Good Samaritan Hospital, Nottingham, MD, USA

Solomon Rojhani, MD Department of Physical Medicine and Rehabilitation, The Johns Hopkins University School of Medicine, Baltimore, MD, USA

Melinda D. Sawyer, MSN, RN, CNS-BC Armstrong Institute for Patient Safety and Quality, John Hopkins University School of Medicine, Baltimore, MD, USA

Stacey L. Schott, MD Department of Internal Medicine, John Hopkins Bayview, Baltimore, MD, USA

Michelle Sharp, MD Department of Pulmonary and Critical Care Medicine, John Hopkins University School of Medicine, Johns Hopkins Hospital, Baltimore, MD, USA

Laura Winner, MBA, RN Armstrong Institute for Patient Safety and Quality, Johns Hopkins Medicine, Baltimore, MD, USA

Benyamin Wise, PharmD Safety Engineer at the Federal Aviation Administration, Washington, DC, USA

Part I
Background to Medical Quality Improvement and Safety

Basic Quality Improvement Terminology

Levi (Levan) Atanelov

Tools

Empathy, physician quality reporting system (PQRS), total quality management (TQM), evidence-based medicine (EBM), continuous quality improvement (CQI), Electronic Medical System (EMR), transparency, systems approach to healthcare, root cause analysis, never events, high-reliability organization (HRO), resilience, Preoccupation with Failure, sensitivity to operations, reluctance to simplify interpretations, deference to expertise

Empathy – the ability to understand and share the feelings of another person.

Physician quality reporting system (PQRS) – a reporting program that uses a combination of incentive payments and payment adjustments to promote reporting of quality information by eligible professionals promoted by the Center of Medicare and Medicaid Services. Providers voluntarily

L. Atanelov (✉)
Department of Physical Medicine and Rehabilitation, Johns Hopkins Hospital, Baltimore, MD, USA
e-mail: leviatanelov@gmail.com

L. Atanelov (ed.), *Resident's Handbook of Medical Quality and Safety*, DOI 10.1007/978-3-319-24190-6_1

provide quality of care-related data on their Medicare patients. Participation in the program is originally encouraged by a financial bonus and later by a financial penalty.

Total quality management (TQM) – all members of the team understand the process and have the tools to improve the process. TQM is a management style. See [1] for more details.

To Err Is Human Institute of Medicine Report – basic conclusion was that national efforts be made to create a mandatory healthcare-related error-reporting system [2].

Crossing the Quality Chiasm Institute of Medicine Report – specific recommendations made to provide healthcare that is safe and consistent in quality, in accord with current scientific evidence (also known as **evidence-based medicine**, EBM), patient centered (i.e., patient values are taken into account strongly), and with no unnecessary time delays [3].

Choosing Wisely Campaign – led by the American Board of Internal Medicine Foundation and aims to improve medical quality by identifying and publicizing interventions that cause overutilization of resources [4]. The initiative is to have different national professional medical organizations identify those interventions that these organizations themselves believe are overutilized and publicize these interventions to their members. See http://www.choosingwisely.org/ for more information.

Continuous quality improvement – quality improvement needs to be a continuous effort to prevent losing the gains made from prior efforts and to adapt to new demands on the system

Accountability – healthcare providers/systems are held responsible for providing quality care with no unnecessary resource utilization. Currently, systems are being created to provide feedback to healthcare organizations and individual providers on their performance compared to expected benchmark standards.

Clinical outcomes – outcomes as defined by patients (e.g. being able to walk again, not having a fever, being able to breathe without the ventilator, not falling anymore) and/or healthcare providers/systems (e.g. resolution of pneumonia, length of hospital stay, patient mortality rate, patient morbidity, medical complications rate, patient falls while on the wards).

Safety – avoiding harm caused to the patients (e.g. hospital-acquired pressure ulcers), their families (e.g. contagious illness like tuberculosis passed on to patient's wife from patient if patient was discharged home without proper precautions), and healthcare system employees (e.g. nurse hurting her back while helping patient get out of bed).

Medical quality – consistently providing care consistent with best standards of medical care, expert medial opinion, and/or patient and family wishes.

Quality improvement project – assesses and/or attempts to bridge the gap between current medical practice and scientifically sound medical care.

Electronic Medical System – electronic software system used to keep track of patient data (e.g. home medication list, past medical history, lab values) and physician entries (physician orders, clinical notes). It can be an important tool in medical quality improvement to monitor trends like compliance with different standards (e.g. documentation of vital signs by nursing) or gather patient-related information like (e.g. hospital length of stay).

Transparency – not hiding problems and mistakes. Overall, the idea is that by hiding problems we lose opportunity to learn from them. This goes as far as admitting to patients when medical errors have been made and asking for apology openly.

The Milgram experiment – this study showed that individuals may allow authority figures to dictate their actions even when these actions starkly oppose their moral stance [5]. Understanding this concept is particularly important in healthcare, as young clinicians may often fall prey to providing care based on outdated practices encouraged by senior physicians, even if this type of care contradicts current standards of quality medical care. Principle of **accountability** means that one is responsible to gently but firmly point out the current evidence to one's seniors in the interest of providing quality medical care, and that failure to do so may possibly have legal consequences. Another lesson to learn from this experiment as it relates to medical quality improvement is that changing the **culture of medicine** is not a simple task, as it may entail having individuals question old and entrenched practices of their authority figures.

Systems approach to healthcare – understanding that when an error is made it is not one individual that is typically at fault but the whole system. For instance, (e.g. if patient got a wrong dose of medication, it could have been that the wrong dose was written by the prescriber and missed by the pharmacy and the nurse; or the nurse gave the wrong medication to the wrong patient in context of being understaffed and having too many difficult patients to care for).

Accountable care organization – healthcare delivery model where reimbursements are tied to quality of medical care provided.

Sentinel event – any unanticipated event in a healthcare setting resulting in death or serious physical or psychological injury to a patient not related to the natural course of the patient's illness. Sentinel events specifically include loss of a limb or gross motor function and any event for which a recurrence would carry a risk of a serious adverse outcome. Sentinel events need to be reported to the JCAHO, an organization that accredits healthcare systems in the USA. Sentinel events can help guide **root cause analysis** (a process to identify the primary causes of the undesirable events) and create preventative practices. **Never events** are a subset of particularly shocking sentinel events, like wrong-side amputation.

Preventative medicine – an ounce of prevention is better than a pound of cure; part of quality medicine is to prevent complications before they occur.

High-reliability organization (HRO) – an organization that avoids significant complications in a complex system with inherent risk factors where accidents are expected. Original lessons from HRO organizations were learned from air traffic control systems, naval aircraft carriers, and nuclear power operations. Part of quality improvement initiatives, it has been suggested that healthcare systems need to become HROs. Five common traits of HROs include [6]:

- **Resilience** – members of the system are prepared to responding when the system failure occurs.
- **Preoccupation with failure** – taking steps to look for any evidence of possible system failures. For instance, when **near-misse** (an event that almost caused an unacceptable outcome) occurs it is seen as a potential weak point of the system.
- **Sensitivity to operations** – constant awareness by the management of the ongoing processes. One way to create this characteristic is to promote more transparency in the organization and make personal observations on the scene.
- **Reluctance to simplify interpretations** – when investigating causes of perceived or real failures, one may have a tendency to accept simplistic explanations, e.g., the physician is bad and made a mistake as opposed to there was inadequate staffing and a lack of error-checking in the system.
- **Deference to expertise** – having a culture where it is acceptable for junior members of the team or those lower on the organizational hierarchy to voice their concerns when they speak based on their expertise (e.g. listening to the janitor that the floor is still too slippery to allow the patient to walk there).

If you have any questions about the information covered in this chapter or other medical safety and quality improvement-related topics, please contact us at http://www.medicalqualityandsafetyforum.com. The website will also provide a forum where you can ask specific questions about your safety and medical quality improvement projects or mentor upcoming medical quality leaders.

References

1. Gustafson D, Hundt A. Findings of innovation research applied to quality management principles for health care. Health Care Manage Rev. 1995;20(2):16–33.

2. Committee on Quality of Healthcare in America, Institute of Medicine, Kohn T, et al. To err is human: building a safer health system. Washington, DC: National Academies Press; 2000.
3. Committee on Quality of Health Care in America, Institute of Medicine. Crossing the quality chiasm: a new health system for the 21st century. Washington, DC: National Academies Press; 2001.
4. Cassel A, Guest A. Choosing wisely – helping physicians and patients make smart decisions about their care. JAMA. 2012; 307(17):1801–2.
5. Milgram S. Behavioral study of obedience. J Abnorm Soc Psychol. 1963;67(4):371–8.
6. Weick K, Sutcliffe K. Managing the unexpected – assuring high performance in an age of complexity. San Francisco: Jossey-Bass; 2001.

History of QI and Safety in the USA

Sina Parizadeh

Tools
IOM, Institute of Medicine of the National Academies, National Quality Forum, National Patient Safety Foundation (NPSF), Accreditation Council for Graduate Medical Education (ACGME), process, structure, outcomes, Joint Commission on Accreditation of Hospitals (JCAH), Institute of Healthcare Improvement (IHI), Quality Interagency Coordination Task Force (QuiC), *To Err Is Human: Building a Safer Health System, Crossing the Quality Chasm: A New Health System for the 21st Century,* Joint Commission on the Accreditation of Healthcare Organizations (JCAHO), Health Resources and Services Administration (HRSA), Centers for Medicare and Medicaid Services (CMS), National Practitioner Database (NPDB), National Committee for Quality Assurance (NCQA)

S. Parizadeh (✉)
Ner Israel Rabbinical College, Baltimore, MD, USA
e-mail: Sinaparizadeh@yahoo.com

L. Atanelov (ed.), *Resident's Handbook of Medical Quality and Safety*, DOI 10.1007/978-3-319-24190-6_2

Quality Improvement (QI) and Patient Safety Definitions

- The IOM, Institute of Medicine of the National Academies, defines *quality* as "the degree to which health services for individuals and populations increase the likelihood of desired health outcomes and are consistent with current professional knowledge" [1].
- *Patient safety* is defined by the National Quality Forum Patient Safety Team as "The prevention and mitigation of harm caused by errors of omission or commission that are associated with healthcare, and involving the establishment of operational systems and processes that minimize the likelihood of errors and maximize the likelihood of intercepting them when they occur" [2].

Who Does QI Concern?

- RESIDENTS: It is a required part of their residency (ACGME will be further increasing emphasis).
- FACULTY: A required part of the ABMS MOC and soon to be a part of MOL (state license).
- EVERYONE INVOLVED IN HEALTHCARE: Nurses, physician assistants, physical therapists, occupational therapists, etc. and even the patients are encouraged and expected to be involved with quality improvement.

Why Is It Important to Emphasize QI?

- Adults receive only half of the clinical services that benefit them.
- Each year, more than 100,000 Americans get the wrong care and are injured as a result [3].
- More than 1.5 million medication errors are made each year [4].
- Healthcare spending has grown from 5 % of GDP in 1960 to about 17 %, or $2.4 trillion, in 2008, nearly half of what the entire world spends on healthcare [5]. The actuaries of the Centers for Medicare and Medicaid Services (CMS) expect healthcare spending will nearly double to $4.4 trillion by 2018 and comprise fully one fifth (20 %) of GDP [6].

- Using the estimates published by the Institute of Medicine (IOM) in 1999, fatal medical errors rank as the 5th to 8th most common cause of death in the USA [3]!
- The range of magnitude of mortality attributed to medical errors was reported by IOM to be 44,000 to 98,000 deaths per year [3]!

Final Decision

- "we have learned to live in a world of mistakes and defective product as if they were necessary for life. It is time to adapt a new philosophy in America." [7]

Dr. Edwards Deming, 1945.

Initial Steps

- In 1910, Dr. *Ernest Codman* proposed the measurement of effectiveness of hospital treatments. "The common sense notion that every hospital should follow every patient it treats, long enough to determine whether or not the treatment has been successful, and then to inquire 'if not, why not?' with a view of preventing similar failures in the future" [8]. He put this idea into practice in Massachusetts General Hospital [9].

Improvements Year by Year

- In 1918, *American College of Surgeons* was founded which developed the minimum standard for the hospitals [10].
- In 1951, Joint Commission on Accreditation of Hospitals **(JCAH)** was established to continue the standardization of the hospitals by providing voluntary accreditation of hospitals based on defined minimum quality standards. This qualification was sought after by the majority of the US hospitals [10].
- In 1966, *Dr. Avedis Donabedian* published "Evaluating the Quality of Medical Care" in which he defined quality of healthcare services and he divided his definition into three parts: **Structure, process** and **outcome**, whereas people before him only focused on the structure of the system

(staffing levels, facility attributes, licensing and accreditation, etc.). [11]

- In 1970, Institute of Medicine **(IOM)** was established by the National Academics of Science to improve the nation's health by providing national advice on issues relating to biomedical science, medicine, and health [12].
- In 1979, six organizations such as American College Health Association, the American Group Practice Association, Federated Ambulatory Surgery Association, etc. joined to found the Accreditation Association for Ambulatory Healthcare **(AAAHC)** to assist ambulatory healthcare organizations and improve the quality of care provided to patients [13].
- In 1991, *Dr. Don Berwick* founded a nonprofit organization under the name of "The Institute of Healthcare Improvement **(IHI)**" to support healthcare changes nationally and worldwide [14].
- In 1997, the National Patient Safety Foundation **(NPSF)** was established to identify new approaches to improving patient safety and call for the innovation necessary to expedite the work. One of the institute's first activities was the publication of an article that identified concepts deemed "as fundamental to the endeavor of achieving meaningful improvement in healthcare system safety"[15].
- In 1998, the Quality Interagency Coordination Task Force (QuiC) was established to enable the participating federal agencies to coordinate their activities to study, measure, and improve the quality of care delivered by federal health programs [16].
- In 1999, the IOM published the famous *To Err Is Human: Building a Safer Health System* where they wrote a report examining the quality of the healthcare. The report concluded that between 44,000 to 98,000 people die each year as a result of preventable medical errors. For comparison, fewer than 50,000 people died of Alzheimer's disease and 17,000 died of illicit drug use in the same year [17]. The following is a quotation of the preface of the book:

> *Errors can be prevented by designing systems that make it hard for people to do the wrong thing and easy for people to do the right thing. Cars are designed so that drivers cannot start them while in reverse because that prevents accidents. Work schedules for pilots are designed so they don't fly too many consecutive hours without rest because alertness and performance are compromised. In health care, building a safer system means designing processes of care to ensure that patients are safe from accidental injury. When agreement has been reached to pursue a course of medical treatment, patients should have the assurance that it will proceed correctly and safely so they have the best chance possible of achieving the desired outcome.* [18]

- In 2001, the IOM published another publication called *Crossing the Quality Chasm: A New Health System for the 21st Century*. This publication showed how the quality of healthcare received by the people of the USA falls short of what it should be and called for potential ways in which change could be implemented in the healthcare system. The push for patient safety that followed the release of these two publications still continues today.
- In 2002, a nonprofit organization under the name of "Joint Commission on the Accreditation of Healthcare Organizations" **(JCAHO)** was established that today (now known as The Joint Commission (TJC)) accredits and certifies more than 20,500 healthcare organizations and programs in the USA. Joint Commission accreditation and certification is recognized nationwide as a symbol of quality that reflects an organization's commitment to meeting certain performance standards [19].

Some of Today's Important Organizations in Healthcare Quality and Safety [20]:

- The Joint Commission on Accreditation of Healthcare Organizations **(JCAHO)**: JCAHO accredits many healthcare organizations including hospitals, ambulatory care facilities, health agencies, and behavioral health services.
- The Health Resources and Services Administration **(HRSA)** is the federal government agency primarily concerned with healthcare.

- The federal government's Centers for Medicare and Medicaid Services **(CMS)** may do site visits to verify that their requirements have been met.
- The National Practitioner Database **(NPDB)** was established through Title IV of Public Law 99–660. The 1986 Healthcare Quality Improvement Act intended to facilitate a comprehensive review of healthcare practitioners' professional credentials.
- The National Committee for Quality Assurance **(NCQA)** works to improve quality of healthcare through accreditation and performance measurement of managed care organizations.
- **URAC**, also known as the American Accreditation HealthCare Commission, is a nonprofit, charitable organization founded to establish standards for the healthcare industry.
- State insurance departments review and seek information about the performance of health providers and insurers.
- **CMS** sets requirements of hospitals and healthcare providers in order to receive payments known as the Conditions of Participation.
- The Institute of Medicine **(IOM)** was established to advance and disseminate scientific knowledge to improve human health.
- The National Quality Forum is a nonprofit organization incorporated to promote a common approach to measuring healthcare quality across national, state, regional, and local groups.

Future

> Between the health care we have and the care we could have lies not just a gap, but a chasm. The American health care delivery system is in need of fundamental change. [21]
>
> *We envision a system of care in which those who give care can boast about their work, and those who receive care can feel total trust and confidence in the care they are receiving.* [22]
>
> *Donald M. Berwick*, MD, MPP
> Chief executive officer of the Institute for Healthcare Improvement

If you have any questions about the information covered in this chapter or other medical safety and quality improvement-related topics, please contact us at http://www.medicalqualityandsafetyforum.com. The website will also provide a forum where you can ask specific questions about your safety and medical quality improvement projects or mentor upcoming medical quality leaders.

References

1. Lohr KN, editor. Medicare: a strategy for quality assurance. Vols I and II. Washington: National Academy Press; 1990.
2. Angood P, Colchamiro E, Lyzenga, A, and Marinelarena M. Meeting of the national quality forum patient safety team. Washington: Unpublished; August 2009.
3. Institute of Medicine (IOM). To err is human: building a safer health system. Washington: National Academies Press; 1999.
4. Institute of Medicine (IOM). Preventing medication errors: quality chasm series. Washington: National Academies Press; 2006.
5. Social Security Advisory Board. The unsustainable cost of health care. Washington: Social Security Advisory Board; 2009.
6. CMS. National health expenditure projections. 2008–2018. https://www.cms.gov/research-statistics-data-and-systems/statistics-trends-and-reports/nationalhealthexpenddata.
7. GAO. Quality management: scoping study.1990. 1:9.
8. Codman EA. The shoulder. Rupture of the supraspinatus tendon and other lesions in or about the sub acromial bursa. Malabar: Kreiger; 1965.
9. Codman EA. A study in hospital efficiency. Terrace: Joint Commission on Accreditation of Healthcare Organizations Oakbrook; 1996.
10. Robert J, Susan B. The AUPHA manual of health services management. Gaithersburg: Aspen Publishers; 1994.
11. Donabedian A. The quality of care: How can it be assessed? JAMA. 1988;121(11):1145–5 0.

12. Edward Berkowitz. To improve human health: a history of the institute of medicine. Washington: National Academy Press; 1998. 2:50.
13. Kongstvedt PR. Essentials of managed health care. Boston: Jones and Bartlett; 2007.
14. Galewitz P. Local hospitals and doctors join forces to improve health care, restrain costs. Kaiser Health News. 2009 and could be found at http://khn.org/news/hospital/Local hospitals and doctors join forces to improve health care, restrain costs.
15. Leape L, Berwick D, Clancy C, Conway J, Gluck P, Guest J, Lawrence D, Morath J, O'Leary D, O'Neill P, Pinakiewicz D, Isaac T. Transforming healthcare: a safety imperative. BMJ Qual saf. 2009;18:424–8.
16. Eisenberg JM, Foster NE, Meyer G, Holland H. Jt Comm J Qual Improv. 2001;27(2):93–100. could be found at http://www.ncbi.nlm.nih.gov/pubmed/11221014.
17. Mokdad A, Marks J, Stroup D, Gerberding J. Actual causes of death in the United States, 2000. JAMA. 2000;291(10):1238–45.
18. Institute of Medicine. To err is human: building a safer health system. Washington: National Academy Press; 1999.
19. Roberts JS, Coale JG, Redman RR. A history of the joint commission on accreditation of hospitals. JAMA. 1987;258(7):936–40.
20. Viswanathan HN, Salmon JW. Accrediting organizations and quality improvement. Am J Manag Care. 2000;6(10):1117–30.
21. Institute of Medicine. Crossing the quality chasm: a new health system for the 21st century. Washington: National Academy Press; 2001.
22. Donald M. Berwick, Institute for Health Care Improvement web site, vision and statement and could be found ar http://www.ihi.org/.

Safety Risk Management Principles from the Federal Aviation Administration

Benyamin Wise

Tools
Bowtie model, preliminary hazard list, functional analysis, Federal Aviation Administration (FAA), safety management system (SMS), safety promotion, safety policy, safety assurance, DIAAT

Safety Risk Management (SRM) (listed but not illustrated)

1. Bowtie model – A model displaying the connection between hazards, causes, and effects. This can aid in determining severity and likelihood of a hazard.
2. Preliminary hazard list (PHL) – A list of initial hazards identified through brainstorming or FA.
3. Functional analysis (FA) – An identification and analysis of the systems functions. Assessing the failure of those functions provides a basis for system hazards.

The Federal Aviation Administration (FAA) provides the safest, most efficient aerospace system in the world. With the

B. Wise (✉)
Safety Engineer at the Federal Aviation Administration, Washington, DC, USA
e-mail: kimbwise@gmail.com

L. Atanelov (ed.), *Resident's Handbook of Medical Quality and Safety*, DOI 10.1007/978-3-319-24190-6_3

adoption of safety management system (SMS), the FAA continues that mission as SMS has become the standard of aviation safety worldwide. SMS provides a repeatable proactive system for addressing safety in the National Airspace System (NAS) by creating a sound safety culture and a means for structured risk identification and decision making.

The FAA's safety management system is built on four pillars:

- Safety promotion – promoting a positive, proactive culture of safety. Examples in the medical field include:
  - Promoting comradery at the workplace
  - Teaching effective communication techniques
  - Encouraging employees to wash hands before and after handling patients
  - Allowing for anyone in the operational hierarchy to update the management when lack of safety is identified anywhere in the system (e.g., "nonpunitive self-reporting"), to encourage mistakes, and therefore hazards, to be identified and addressed instead of hidden
  - Encouraging the following operational guidelines:
- Safety policy – the rules outlining the requirements of safety within the organization.
- Safety risk management (SRM) – the process by which a system is analyzed for safety.
- Safety assurance (SA) – the process of reviewing and updating the results of SRM, i.e., monitoring one or several key variables identified by SRM for a desired time interval to ensure that the gains established during the SRM persist. This is similar to the control phase of DMAIC.

SRM and SA form the core of SMS, while safety promotion and policy support SRM and SA.

This chapter will focus on SRM. The SRM process follows five steps, of which the acronym is DIAAT.

1. Describe the system.
   (a) Allows one to properly scope and assess the problem
   (b) There are many techniques to do this. One popular method is called the 5 m model.
      - Machine – hardware, software, and human interaction
      - (Hu)man – operators and maintenance personnel
      - Media – environment system operates in
      - Mission – functions the system needs to perform
      - Management – procedures and policy governing the system
2. Identify the hazards.
   (a) Identifying what can go wrong/fail.
   (b) This process starts with collecting all ideas of potential hazards.
   (c) Once that is complete, a second assessment of the hazards can be done to remove redundant or incorrect (causes/effects) hazards.
3. Analyze the hazard.
   (a) Analyze the severity (1–5) of each hazard effect (undesirable outcome).
   (b) Analyze the likelihood (A–E) of each effect by assessing the likelihood of both the hazard causes and effects.
   (c) It's important to analyze the severity first. Otherwise, the likelihood will color one's assessment of the severity.
4. Assess the risk.
   (a) A combination of severity and likelihood that classifies a hazard as high (red), medium (yellow), or low (green) risk.
   (b) High risk is unacceptable, medium risk is acceptable but mitigation is recommended, and low risk is acceptable without mitigation (Table 1).

	5	4	3	2	1
A					
B					
C					
D					
E					*

* No single point failure permitted

TABLE 1 Risk Matrix

5. Treat the risk.
   (a) Identify mitigations (e.g., revising system design, modifying procedures)
   (b) Develop risk-treatment plan
   (c) Develop risk-monitoring plan
   (d) Implementing and verifying mitigations

SRM Example

As a simple example, consider a scenario of ice forming on a sidewalk. Potential causes could be faulty sidewalk design and lack of salting procedures during rain and freezing temperatures. The hazard would be the ice forming on a sidewalk. The effects would include someone slipping and breaking something. Various outcomes (effects) can be assessed for severity and likelihood using questions such as "What's the worst outcome?" "How likely is that?" and "What mitigations exist?" If the hazard is determined to be high, additional mitigation would need to be put in place (i.e., safer sidewalk design, better procedures, etc.) and monitored.

If you have any questions about the information covered in this chapter or other medical safety and quality improvement-related topics, please contact us at http://www.medicalqualityandsafetyforum.com. The website will also provide a forum where you can ask specific questions about your safety and medical quality improvement projects or mentor upcoming medical quality leaders.

Human Factors Engineering for Quality Improvement and Research in Health Care

Ayse P. Gurses

> **Tools**
> Cognitive walk-through, contextual inquiry, focus groups, heuristic analysis, interviews, prototyping, questionnaires and surveys, the Systems Engineering Initiative for Patient Safety model, task analysis, time and motion studies, and usability evaluation, physical ergonomics, cognitive ergonomics, microergonomics, work system, process, outcomes

Definition

Human factors engineering (HFE) is "the scientific discipline concerned with the understanding of interactions among humans and other elements of a system, and the profession that applies theory, principles, data and methods to design in order to optimize human well-being and overall system performance"(http://www.iea.cc/whats/index.html).

A.P. Gurses (✉)
Hopkins Bloomberg School of Public Health, Baltimore, MD, USA

Department of Anesthesiology and Critical Medicine,
Johns Hopkins Hospital, Baltimore, MD, USA
e-mail: agurses1@jhmi.edu

L. Atanelov (ed.), *Resident's Handbook of Medical Quality and Safety*, DOI 10.1007/978-3-319-24190-6_4

Domains of Specialization Within HFE

There are three sub-domains within the discipline of HFE: physical ergonomics, cognitive ergonomics, and macroergonomics [1].

- *Physical ergonomics* focuses on how to (re)design physical environments (e.g., physical layout of an intensive care unit) or tools (e.g., ergonomics and design of laparoscopic surgery instruments) to improve human performance.
- *Cognitive ergonomics* develops solutions to improve overall system performance considering the cognitive abilities and limitations (e.g., limitations in working memory and attention) of human beings. Common areas of focus under this sub-domain include better management of mental workload, improvement of decision-making, enhancement of human-computer interaction, and development of effective training programs.
- *Macroergonomics* uses a variety of HFE tools and methods to (re)design the overall work system, taking into account the interactions and fit between different system components. Enhancing teamwork and coordination, improving safety culture, and redesigning jobs (e.g., scheduling breaks, changing the duration of shifts) are examples of improvement efforts that can benefit from macroergonomics.

Conceptual Model to Guide Health-Care Quality Improvement and Research Efforts

According to the Systems Engineering Initiative for Patient Safety (SEIPS) model (Fig. 1), a human factors engineering model of quality and safety of care, the performance and outcomes (e.g., readmission rates, health-care acquired infections) in any health-care organization, depends on the design of the work system (structure) and the related processes

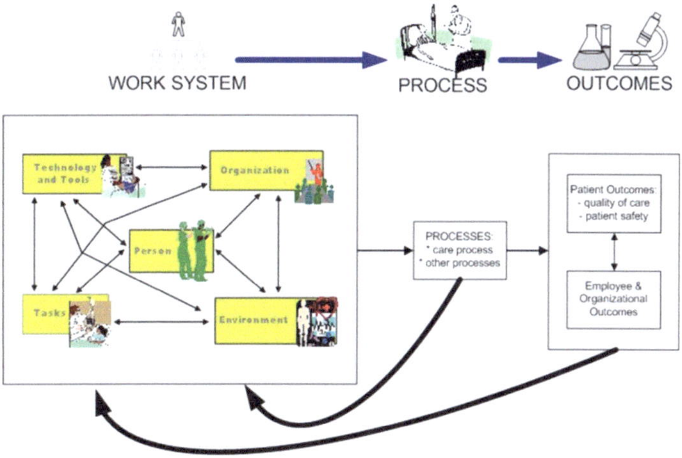

FIG. 1 Systems Engineering Initiative for Patient Safety (SEIPS) model (Carayon et al. [2], p. i51)

(both care processes and other processes). HFE experts study the interactions between individuals and elements of the work system in which they work including physical environment, tasks, tools and technologies, teamwork, and organizational environment. They then develop solutions (i.e., redesigning particular aspects of the work system) while systematically considering the interactions among different work system elements to avoid any potential unanticipated negative impact of the proposed solutions [2].

Human Factors Engineering Methods

Human factors engineers use a variety of qualitative (e.g., interviews, focus groups) and quantitative methods (e.g., questionnaire, time and motion studies) for data collection and analysis. A sample list of these methods is given in Table 1. It is important to note that Table 1 provides descriptions of only a very small subset method; interested readers are

TABLE 1 A sample list of methods and tools used in human factors engineering

Method/ Tool name	Definition	Abbreviated example
Cognitive walk-through	A step-by-step process of having the users talk about their thinking and action-taking process while performing specific predefined tasks. It can be done while the users are performing or after they completed performing the task. A very common cognitive-walk-through method is think-aloud, where the users talk about their thinking process while they perform the tasks. As medical workflows involve multiple processes, walk-throughs can be especially useful in determining user cognitive processes to better multiple systems	The physicians being asked to explain their thinking while accessing a specific lab value of a patient through the electronic health record
Contextual inquiry	Unobtrusive observation of users performing relevant tasks in their natural working environments, coupled with short questioning	A physician is observed while performing her duties in the ICU and is asked short questions about the tasks she is performing
Heuristic analysis	Involves the evaluation by clinical and/or human factors/ usability engineering experts of the technology in how it conforms to human factors/usability rules	A team of human factors experts determining and comparing different brands of medical devices in terms of their design and usability before a purchasing decision is made

Interviews	Systematic and in-depth data gathering regarding a topic/focus area by asking detailed questions. Interviews can be structured (a strict set of questions), semi-structured (a few open-ended questions coupled with specific probes), and/or unstructured (no previously determined set of questions)	Physicians and nurses being interviewed about their most commonly encountered problems involving the physical layout and design in their unit
Prototyping	Developing a simple representation of a new design alternative (e.g., information technology, medical device, physical layout) and its components through rapidly developed, inexpensive models, which, in most cases, are not fully functional but fulfill the needs of the testing for functionality purposes. Multiple prototypes can be developed to simulate the new design alternatives, and simulations can be used to better understand the functionalities and common scenarios	Developing a mock-up of user interfaces of a critical component of an electronic health record system for experimentation with physicians and nurses
Questionnaires and surveys	Written questions and surveys allow relevant opinion and information collection regarding various work system elements. They can also be very useful in evaluating the impact of an intervention on the work system, processes, and outcomes. Surveys can be administered in person, via postal mail, on the phone, and online	Surveying patients and family members for their opinions regarding the redesigned hospital discharge process

(continued)

Table 1 (continued)

Method/ Tool name	Definition	Abbreviated example
Task analysis	Systematic methods to produce detailed descriptions of tasks and their corresponding sub-activities	Determining which exact tasks are repetitively done in an ICU by a nurse, how long each task and subtask lasts, and work-arounds and potential risks associated with each task
Time and motion studies	Determining the exact typical motion and the typical time it takes to complete a task and its components correspond to time and motion studies. Video recording the tasks and using stopwatch are common activities accompanying time and motion studies	Using time and motion analysis to determine what percentage of nursing time is spent on direct patient care and indirect patient care (e.g., walking in the unit, documentation)
Usability evaluation	Involves understanding the exact nature of interactions between users and technologies	Laboratory testing of a newly developed information technology

encouraged to consult other resources (e.g., [3]) to learn more about the HFE methods.

Application Domains

Human Factors Engineering can be used in almost all aspects of health-care quality improvement efforts (See [4] for detailed examples). Some examples of the use of HFE in health care are listed below:

- To reduce health-care acquired infections through work system redesign such as standardization, reducing ambiguity in systems [5], and improving culture of safety
- To assess risks associated with a new electronic health record system implementation proactively (before implementation) and to develop appropriate strategies with the purpose of mitigating these risks
- To conduct effective root cause analysis and medical-error accident investigations for creating more effective learning organizations
- To evaluate and compare different brands of medical devices from a usability point of view in order to inform purchasing decisions
- To improve care coordination and teamwork among clinicians
- To identify patient and family member needs and to develop solutions for increasing the patient and family centeredness of care

If you have any questions about the information covered in this chapter or other medical safety and quality improvement-related topics, please contact us at http://www.medicalqualityandsafetyforum.com. The website will also provide a forum where you can ask specific questions about your safety and medical quality improvement projects or mentor upcoming medical quality leaders.

References

1. Gurses AP, Ozok AA, Pronovost PJ. Time to accelerate integration of human factors and ergonomics in patient safety. BMJ Qual Saf. 2011;21(4):347–51.
2. Carayon P, Hundt AS, Karsh B-T, Gurses AP, Alvarado CJ, Smith M, Brennan PF. Work system design for patient safety: the SEIPS model. Qual Saf Health Care. 2006;15 Suppl 1:i50–8.
3. Stanton NA, Salmon PM, Rafferty LA, Walker GH, Baber C, Jenkins DP. Human factors methods: a practical guide for engineering and design. 2nd ed. Burlington: Ashgate Publishing; 2013.
4. Carayon P. Handbook of human factors and ergonomics in health care and patient safety. Boca Raton: CRC Press; 2011.
5. Gurses AP, Seidl K, Vaidya V, Bochicchio G, Harris A, Hebden J, Xiao Y. Systems ambiguity and guideline compliance: a qualitative study of how intensive care units follow evidence-based guidelines to reduce healthcare-associated infections. Qual Saf Health Care. 2008;17(5):351–9.

The Role of Informatics and Electronic Health Record in Current Medical Practice: What Are the Benefits of Medical Informatics to the Clinician?

Andre Cassell

Tools
Electronic Health Record (EHR), clinical informatics, data mining, Stata, R, SAS, Microsoft Excel, data analysis, data sets

What Are Electronic Health Records

President Bush in 2004 put forth the goal that every American would have an electronic health record by 2014 [1]. The impetus behind the aggressive carryover of records to electronic form stemmed from trying to fix inefficiencies in the hospital

A. Cassell (✉)
Department of Physical Medicine and Rehabilitation, John Hopkins Hospital, 600 North Wolfe Street, Suite 160, Baltimore, MD 21287, USA
e-mail: acassel5@jhmi.edu

L. Atanelov (ed.), *Resident's Handbook of Medical Quality and Safety*, DOI 10.1007/978-3-319-24190-6_5

and improve quality. Quality improvement, reduction of errors, and fixing systems within hospitals were seen as potential ways to decrease the cost of healthcare in the United States. Medicare and Medicaid currently have incentive programs for EHR [2].

The literature up till this point suggests that electronic health record (EHR) is not well defined; EHR has many functions and many types of data [3]. Based on the International Standardizations Organization, EHR is a "repository of patient data in digital form, stored and exchanged securely, and accessible by multiple authorized users."

Research and Data Mining

"Health informatics is an evolving specialization that links information technology, communications and healthcare to improve the quality and safety of patient care" [4]. The accessibility of EHR makes it possible for researchers to answer questions involving quality improvement and/or outcomes of an intervention. For small sets of data where sets of populations are being used and the data is relatively refined (i.e., comparing significant differences in blood pressure in a prospective, randomized controlled trial), excel and SAS are great tools to calculate significant differences between groups. Features are built in within these programs to be able to run t-tests and even evaluate differences of means in nonparametric data. In medicine, however, not all data for the purposes of answering complex clinical data are as clean. Programming languages like Stata and R are useful in this regard and are instrumental in the field of informatics. Stata and R allow for multivariate analysis, analyzing data on a subset of patients that have certain characteristics, and allow for easier graphical interpretation by a few lines of code. Such clinical questions could look like the following:

- For patients under 50 years of age, what was the first and last hemoglobin A1c for the June 2014 to September 2014 time period?

- From all patients in the hospital who have been transferred to rehab from a medicine floor in the past year with a diagnosis of spinal cord injury and under 60 years of age, run a multivariate analysis for mobility scores.

The use of programming languages and software to come up with outcomes to complex clinical questions is extremely relevant when it comes to quality improvement both on a nationwide scale and on the individual hospital scale.

Hospital-Based EHR and Ways to Analyze Outcomes

A potential benefit of informatics and data analysis comes from being able to provide the clinician with an answer to a clinical problem specific to the clinician's patients. Many of the platforms being used today within institutions including EPIC and Cerner have an option to trend laboratory data, blood glucose, and other lab parameters over a certain time period. These platforms, however, do not provide the clinician to select out the African American patients under 50 years of age, or trend the LDL from right before a statin was given till three months after, or other ways to "subset" the data. This is an added benefit of medical informatics – to be able to engineer software to provide the clinician with answers to complicated questions about his or her patients.

To be able to perform these operations in an EHR is somewhat difficult, as different clinicians will want to answer different questions and will need different parameters to be recorded on the same platform. EPIC Systems currently has a physician builder course that teaches physicians how to build features into EPIC for the use of analyzing outcomes and trending specific data. These physicians must work in conjunction with analysts within their hospital for their specific ideas to come to fruition. Improvements in outcomes are especially important to the individual physician as hospitals and institutions are penalized for poor outcomes.

Conclusion

EHR offers the physician the opportunity to study large and small populations of data, within institution and across institutions. Furthermore, for the physicians who want to track the laboratory data, vital signs, missed appointments, or other clinically relevant data with patients under their practice, informatics represents a developing and exciting field that can make this endeavor feasible.

If you have any questions about the information covered in this chapter or other medical safety and quality improvement-related topics, please contact us at http://www.medicalqualityandsafetyforum.com. The website will also provide a forum where you can ask specific questions about your safety and medical quality improvement projects or mentor upcoming medical quality leaders.

References

1. Simborg W. Promoting electronic health record adoption. is it the correct focus? J Am Med Inform Assoc. 2008;15(2):127–9. doi:DOI:10.1197/jamia.M2573.
2. EHR Incentive programs. (n.d.). Retrieved 30 Dec 2014, from http://www.cms.gov/Regulations-and Guidance/Legislation/EHRIncentivePrograms/index.html?redirect=/EHRIncentivePrograms/
3. Häyrinen K et al. Definition, structure, content, use and impacts of electronic health records: a review of the research literature. Int J Med Inform. 2008;77(5):291–304.
4. What is health informatics? (n.d.). Retrieved 30 Dec 2014 from http://www.usfhealthonline.com/resources/healthcare/what-is-health-informatics/#.VKJSB8ACA

Part II
Perspectives for Residency Program Directors and Hospital Administration

The Importance of Resident Involvement in Quality Improvement: An Investment in Our Future

Redonda G. Miller

> **Tools**
> HPSQC, Accreditation Council for Graduate Medical Education (ACGME), Clinical Learning Environment Review (CLER) Program

As frontline providers of patient care, residents are key drivers of quality at academic medical centers. Therefore, it is essential for teaching hospitals to engage their residents as core participants in organizational initiatives to improve the quality of patient care. Simply put, the success of an academic medical center's quality improvement programs is dependent on the participation of residents.

Prior to 2008, there is a scant literature describing residents' participation in quality improvement initiatives [1]. While the quality movement in health care took root several decades ago, the imperative to involve residents in efforts to improve patient

R.G. Miller
Department of Medical Affairs, The John Hopkins Hospital,
600 North Wolfe Street, Billing Administration 125B, Balitmore,
MD 21287, USA
e-mail: rgmiller@jhmi.edu

L. Atanelov (ed.), *Resident's Handbook of Medical Quality and Safety*, DOI 10.1007/978-3-319-24190-6_6

care is just now gaining ground. This imperative has largely been driven by Accreditation Council for Graduate Medical Education (ACGME) program requirements.

A key milestone occurred in 2011 when the ACGME established the Clinical Learning Environment Review (CLER) Program. One of CLER's six areas of focus is quality improvement, including "how sponsoring institutions engage residents in the use of data to improve systems of care, reduce health-care disparities, and improve patient outcomes" [2]. Also in 2011, revised ACGME program requirements added emphasis on active resident involvement in quality improvement [3, 4]. More recently, revised ACGME institutional requirements implemented in 2014 explicitly call for residents to have an active role in quality initiatives [5].

While engaging residents in institutional quality initiatives fulfills ACGME requirements, the rewards are more far-reaching. By participating in quality projects, residents gain invaluable leadership experience, while at the same time helping to solve problems for the institution and enhancing the quality of care for patients. Furthermore, it has been shown that involving residents in quality initiatives that permit them to witness patient care improvements is a more powerful form of education than classroom quality improvement theory [6]. Importantly, trainees reap the fulfillment that comes with solving a problem and developing the tools to provide quality patient care that they will carry with them throughout their career [7].

To engage housestaff in quality at the Johns Hopkins Hospital, a group of residents partnered with hospital leadership to develop the Housestaff Patient Safety and Quality Council (HPSQC) in 2012. Modeled after the successful Housestaff Quality Council established in New York-Presbyterian Hospital/Weill Cornell Medical Center, HPSQC provides a forum where residents can share their experiences on improving quality and receive valuable feedback. The goals of the HPSQC are to incorporate residents into the hospital's quality improvement structure and to build capacity among our trainees, with the ultimate objectives of improving patient care and creating an organizational culture that promotes greater house staff engagement. The HPSQC is run by residents under the direction of a self-created charter. It is sanctioned by our Medical Executive Committee and established as a medical staff committee in our bylaws. The HPSQC is further supported by a leadership cabinet of faculty champions and hospital administrator advocates.

During the preliminary meetings of the Housestaff Patient Safety and Quality Council, the energy and enthusiasm in the room were palpable. Because of the residents' unique frontline position, many of them conveyed a thoughtful understanding of the day-to-day problems and already had ideas for making improvements. Furthermore, they were grateful for the opportunity to share their perceptions. It soon became apparent that our residents would bring a new perspective to situations that more senior physicians might take for granted and that the time was clearly right for engaging our residents as partners in our institutional quality efforts.

As part of their HPSQC membership, Johns Hopkins residents are taking on exciting projects that align institutional quality goals with residency training goals. During the HPSQC's inaugural year, a resident-driven interdisciplinary initiative helped to increase inpatient influenza and pneumococcal vaccination rates. The following year, a second project was designed to improve the quality and timeliness of inpatient discharges.

There are numerous quality projects that residents can tackle successfully, provided they are awarded the necessary time, resources, and mentorship [7]. Ultimately, the fruits of these efforts create a win-win situation for all – the trainees, the institution, our patients, and, in short, the culture of medicine. While learning to address significant quality issues for the institution, our residents will become stewards of high-quality patient care and future leaders in safety and quality. This is a critical and wise investment in our future.

If you have any questions about the information covered in this chapter or other medical safety and quality improvement-related topics, please contact us at http://www.medicalqualityandsafetyforum.com. The website will also provide a forum where you can ask specific questions about your safety and medical quality improvement projects or mentor upcoming medical quality leaders.

References

1. Patow CA, Karpovich K, Riesenberg LA, et al. Residents' engagement in quality improvement: a systematic review of the literature. Acad Med. 2009;84(12):1757–64.
2. Accreditation Council for Graduate Medical Education. Clinical Learning Environment (CLER) Program. Available at: http://www.acgme.org/acgmeweb/tabid/436/ProgramandInstitutionalAccreditation/NextAccreditationSystem/ClinicalLearningEnvironmentReviewProgram.aspx. Accessed 24 Oct 2014.
3. Accreditation Council for Graduate Medical Education. Common program requirements. Available at: http://www.acgme.org/acgmeweb/Portals/0/PDFs/Common_Program_Requirements_07012011[2].pdf Accessed 24 Oct, 2014.
4. Philibert I, Gonzalez J, Lannon C, Lieh-Lai M, et al. Quality improvement skills for pediatric residents: from lecture to implementation and sustainability. Acad Pediatr. 2014;14(1):40–6.
5. Accreditation Council for Graduate Medical Education. Institutional Requirements, July 1, 2014. Available at: https://www.acgme.org/acgmeweb/Portals/0/InstitutionalRequirements_07012014.pd Accessed 24 Oct 2014.
6. Philibert I. Involving residents in quality improvement: contrasting "top-down" and bottom-up approaches-IHI 90 day project. Chicago: Accreditation Council for Graduate Medical Education; 2008.
7. Hawkins CM, Nagy P. Quality improvement projects for residents. J Am Coll Radiol. 2013 Apr;10(4):301–2. doi:10.1016/j.jacr.2012.12.022.

Residency Program Director's Perspective on Patient Safety and Quality Improvement

R. Samuel Mayer

> **Tools**
> Accreditation Council for Graduate Medical Education (ACGME), Clinical Learning Environment Review (CLER) Program, patient safety, quality improvement, transitions in care, supervision, duty hour oversight, fatigue management and mitigation

My Story

I have been deeply involved in quality improvement and patient safety for over 15 years. I have been our department's deputy director for quality improvement from 2001 to 2013. But an episode that occurred about 10 years truly engaged me passionately in this area:

> A 22 year old man came to our hospital for resection of a benign cervical spinal cord tumor. He was subsequently transferred to our inpatient rehabilitation unit for therapy of his incomplete tetraparesis, where I was the attending physician. He had been making

R.S. Mayer (✉)
Department of Physical Medicine and Rehabilitation,
Johns Hopkins University School of Medicine, 600 Wolfe Street,
Phipps #198, Baltimore, MD 21287, USA
e-mail: rmayer2@jhmi.edu

L. Atanelov (ed.), *Resident's Handbook of Medical Quality and Safety*, DOI 10.1007/978-3-319-24190-6_7

progress to the point of being able to eat pizza using his own hands. Over the weekend his parents saw small declines in his abilities but nothing defining. Was he just too tired from therapy to now hold his own pizza or was something happening? The team decided to just watch him for the rest of the weekend. There were no frank neurologic changes. By late Monday he became a complete tetraplegic and an emergent CT scan showed a bleed into his previous OR site. He was emergently transferred to the neuro critical unit where he was put on life support. I met with the family who were understandably anguished and angry. It was one of the most difficult conversations of my career. The family felt as though we just did not listen to them when they saw and reported all the subtle changes in their son's condition, and they were right. Later that week the parents withdrew care and he soon died.

Why Program Directors Should Care About Patient Safety and Quality Improvement

Anyone who touches health care in any way should care about patient safety and quality improvement. This goes for everyone from the hospital environmental service technician to the CEO of a pharmaceutical company. It applies to nurses and rehabilitation therapists, social workers, and psychologists. Every member of the health-care team needs to be actively involved in providing safe, effective, and efficient high-quality care. Pronovost et al. tell us "To improve, caregivers need to know what to do, how they are doing, and be able to improve the processes of care" [1] and that care must focus on the most important stakeholders in the system: patients and their families. This is why we went into the health-care professions to begin with, and we should never forget that.

Physicians, in particular, play a critical role in ensuring safe, high-quality care. Doctors are often not the most important members of the health-care team. For better or worse, however, most stakeholders view them as the team leaders [2, 3]. Schwartz and Pogge point out, "Although most physicians possess the traits essential for leadership, the vast majority lacks the technical skills necessary for major leadership/management roles that will both change and empower the local healthcare service delivery environment. Such skills include strategic and tactical planning, persuasive communication, negotiation, financial decision-making, team building, conflict resolution, and interviewing" [3]. Furthermore, for quality improvement, analytic skills are essential [4]. As residency program directors, it is incumbent upon us to teach these skills to our trainees.

Our hospitals, which generally pay our residents' salaries, now have a keen financial interest in these issues, if they weren't already part of their mission. Under new Medicare reimbursement rules, about 1500 hospitals were penalized in 2013 for poor-quality outcomes [5].

As if the above were not adequate reasons for getting program directors' attention, the Accreditation Council on Graduate Medical Education has issued new institutional and common program requirements which mandate resident involvement in quality improvement and patient safety [6]. The requirements, encompassed under the Clinical Learning Environment Review (CLER), are as follows:

CLER assesses sponsoring institutions in the following six focus areas:

- ***Patient safety*** *– including opportunities for residents to report errors, unsafe conditions, and near misses and to participate in inter-professional teams to promote and enhance safe care.*
- ***Quality improvement*** *– including how sponsoring institutions engage residents in the use of data to improve systems of care, reduce health-care disparities, and improve patient outcomes.*
- ***Transitions in care*** *– including how sponsoring institutions demonstrate effective standardization and oversight of transitions of care.*
- ***Supervision*** *– including how sponsoring institutions maintain and oversee policies of supervision concordant with ACGME requirements in an environment at both the institutional and program level that assures the absence of retribution.*
- ***Duty hours oversight, fatigue management, and mitigation*** *– including how sponsoring institutions (i) demonstrate effective and meaningful oversight of duty hours across all residency programs institution-wide, (ii) design systems and provide settings that facilitate fatigue management and*

mitigation, and (iii) provide effective education of faculty members and residents in sleep, fatigue recognition, and fatigue mitigation.

- ***Professionalism** – with regard to how sponsoring institutions educate for professionalism, monitor behavior on the part of residents and faculty, and respond to issues concerning (i) accurate reporting of program information, (ii) integrity in fulfilling educational and professional responsibilities, and (iii) veracity in scholarly pursuits.*

Why Residency Program Directors Should Own This Book

The Resident Manual for Patient Safety and Quality Improvement is written primarily *by residents for residents.* However, I believe it also belongs on every program director's bookshelf. It provides substantial information about patient safety and quality improvement and demystifies the processes of culture change, program development, and analytics. It provides examples of practical ideas to engage your residents in patient safety and quality improvement projects.

Establishing a Culture of Safety

The residency program director's first and foremost responsibility is to promote a culture of safety. This responsibility cannot fall on the program director's shoulders alone. Upper management in both the institution and the department must make this a primary priority, of course. Perhaps more importantly each faculty member, resident, and staff member within the department must buy into this framework. Each team member must be educated on the critical importance of patient safety and quality improvement upon orientation as a new employee, and at regular intervals thereafter. All departmental staff meetings should have patient safety as an agenda item.

Hopefully, your institution measures the climate of safety with regular (at least annual) surveys such as the Safety

Attitudes Questionnaire™ [7]. If not, as a program director, you can certainly survey your own residents and faculty. Regular feedback on results can at least start the conversation.

There are a number of ways to improve the culture once this baseline is established [8]. These include:

- *Encourage residents to report incidents of potential harm.*
- *Do inter-professional training sessions with residents and staff on communication and teamwork.*
- *Establish a house staff quality improvement council, and have resident representatives on your departmental quality improvement committee.*
- *Hold resident didactic sessions on quality improvement methodologies and analytics.*
- *Have each resident participate in a quality improvement project.*
- *Revise morbidity and mortality conferences.*
- *Hold residents accountable for participation in quality improvement in their milestone assessments.*

Resident Reporting of Incidents

Without prompting and education, residents rarely report adverse events. At Oregon Health and Science University, only 1.6 % of adverse event reports institutionally were initiated by residents. After an intensive educational campaign, including the provision of incentives, that increased to 9.6 % [9]. Empowering residents to report actual harmful events and – perhaps more importantly – events which are potentially harmful is a great first step to engaging them in a culture of safety.

Teamwork and Communication

Improved communication is essential to safe patient care. Issues of communication and teamwork were identified as root causes in 563 of 887 sentinel events reported to The Joint Commission by health-care organizations accredited by that body [10]. We believe that inter-professional training in teamwork should be mandatory for all graduate medical education programs. We do a half-day required training session for our residents and departmental staff in nursing, rehabilitation therapy services, psychology, and social work. We have customized our training to meet the specialized needs of physical medicine and rehabilitation; other departments at Johns Hopkins have also developed programs customized to their specialties. These sessions include real-life stories such as the opening paragraph of this chapter. The participants engage in role-playing activities, often swapping roles to further understand other health professionals' viewpoints.

Establish a House Staff Quality Council

A number of institutions have established house staff quality councils based on the model developed at New York-Presbyterian Hospital/Weill Cornell Medical Center [11]. Residents from every department meet regularly with senior hospital management (e.g., Vice President for Medical Affairs or Chief Safety Officer) and work on multidisciplinary action plans based on resident-identified harms or institutional safety dashboard concerns. Talk to your graduate medical education committee about forming one.

Didactic Education

Often departmental faculty have not received sufficient training in quality improvement methodology, so the program director should identify a few core faculty who are willing and able to receive basic training in this. The program director should also identify institutional resources for this. Institutional resources can be supplemented with online training programs as well. The Institute for Healthcare Improvement (IHI) has series of open enrollment courses free to faculty and residents [12]. Decide what level of training is appropriate for your residents, but mandate that they at least receive a basic minimum. In addition, you will hopefully engage some residents to seek more advanced training. The Armstrong Institute on Patient Safety and Quality Care at Johns Hopkins, for example, offers various levels of training for residents and fellows.

Participation in Quality Improvement Projects

Didactics are important, but do not substitute for experiential education. We require each of our residents to participate in a quality improvement project. There are at least three models of types of projects for residents:

- ***Team-based model*** – *focused on behavior change and limited process change to improve a workflow that is within the control of the interdisciplinary medical team*
- ***Unit-based model*** – *focused on a workflow in a particular unit or clinic with aims that are tied to institutional priorities*
- ***Systems-based model*** – *focused on a workflow that crosses multiple units/clinics with an aim to improve systems at the departmental or institutional level*

These can vary considerably in time frames and level of individual resident commitment required.

Death to Morbidity and Mortality Conferences

Traditional morbidity and mortality (M&M) conferences often degenerate into "shame and blame" sessions. These are counterproductive and can devastate a culture of safety, where residents feel empowered to report harmful situations. Sometimes, in order to skirt the "shame and blame" scenarios, residents will use these to present esoteric cases so that they can self-congratulate themselves on making a rare diagnosis. Others will use the opportunity to lay blame on people or departments not present at the conference. This does little to promote safety.

We have revised our departmental M&M conference, renaming it patient safety and quality rounds. Each month, the presenting resident reviews an item from our departmental safety dashboard. The resident first presents an example of a patient harmed by the problem identified on the dashboard. Then the criteria used (inclusions and exclusion criteria, numerators and denominators), baseline performance and current data trends, and projects in place to correct deficiencies are presented. A lively discussion about next steps ensues. This engages all of our residents to work on departmentally identified quality goals.

Hold Residents Accountable

We must not conflate systems-based thinking in root cause analysis of medical error with a "no-blame" environment [13]. Poorly performing residents do need to be held accountable for errors made because of lack of following policies (e.g., not practicing hand hygiene) or not seeking appropriate help when needed [14]. We orient our residents on day one that they will never be disciplined for calling for help or asking a "silly" question. However, they may get in serious trouble if they fail to ask for assistance in situations in which they were "over their heads." The program director must assure that adequate supervision is always available and that if those resources are not accessed, residents hold some responsibility.

If you have any questions about the information covered in this chapter or other medical safety and quality improvement-related topics, please contact us at http://www.medicalqualityandsafetyforum.com. The website will also provide a forum where you can ask specific questions about your safety and medical quality improvement projects or mentor upcoming medical quality leaders.

References

1. Pronovost PJ, Nolan T, Zieger S, Rubin H. How can clinicians measure safety and quality in acute care? Lancet. 2004;363(9414):1061–7.
2. Romano CA, Pangaro LN. What is a doctor and what is a nurse? A perspective for future practice and education. Acad Med. 2013;89(7):970–2.
3. Schwartz RW, Pogge C. Physician leadership: essential skills in a changing environment. Am J Surg. 2000;180(3):187–92.
4. Pronovost PJ, Goeschell CA, Marstell JA, Sexton JB, Pham JC, Berenholz SM. Framework for patient safety research and improvement. Circulation. 2009;119:330–7.
5. Nearly 1,500 hospitals penalized under medical program rating quality. [Internet]: Kaiser Health News; 2013 [updated November 14, 2013; cited October 10, 2014]. Available from: http://www.kaiserhealthnews.org/stories/2013/november/14/value-based-purchasing-medicare.aspx http://findit.library.jhu.edu/resolve?sid=Refworks%3AJohns%20Hopkins%20Institution&charset=utf-8&__char_set=utf8&genre=article&date=2013&atitle=Nearly%201%2C500%20Hospitals%20Penalized%20Under%20Medical%20Program%20Rating%20Quality.&
6. Clinical learning environment review (CLER) program [Internet]. Chicago: Accreditation Council on Graduate Medical Education; 2014 [cited October 10, 2014]. Available from: http://www.acgme.org/acgmeweb/tabid/436/ProgramandInstitutionalAccreditation/NextAccreditationSystem/ClinicalLearningEnvironmentReviewProgram.aspx http://findit.library.jhu.edu/resolve?sid=Refworks%3AJohns%20Hopkins%20Institution&charset=utf-8&__char_set=utf8&genre=article&date=2014&atitle=Clinical%20Learning%20Environment%20Review%20(CLER)%20Program&
7. Sexton JB, Heinrich RL, Neilands TB, et al. The safety attitudes questionnaire: psychometric properties benchmarking data, and emerging research. BMC Health Serv Res. 2006;6:44–54.
8. Paine LA, Rosenstein BJ, Sexton JB, Kent P, Holzmueller CG, Pronovost PJ. Assessing and improving safety culture throughout an academic medical centre: a prospective cohort study. Qual Saf Health Care. 2010;19:547–54.
9. Scott DR, Weimer M, English C, et al. A novel approach to increase residents' involvement in reporting adverse events. Acad

Med [increased resident reports 1% to 9% of hosp incident reports]. 2011;86(6):742–6.
10. Sentinel event type by year 1195–2013 [Internet]. Oak Brook: The Joint Commision; 2014 [cited 10/14/14]. Available from: http://www.jointcommission.org/assets/1/18/Event_Type_by_Year_1995-2Q_2014.pdf http://findit.library.jhu.edu/resolve?sid=Refworks%3AJohns%20Hopkins%20Institution&charset=utf-8&__char_set=utf8&genre=article&aulast=The%20Joint%20Commission&date=2014&atitle=Sentinel%20Event%20Type%20by%20Year%201195-2013&au=The%20Joint%20Commission%20&
11. Fleischut P, Faggiani S, Evans A, et al. The effect of a novel housestaff quality council on quality and patient safety. Jt Comm J Qual Patient Saf. 2012;38(7):311–7.
12. IHI open school [Internet]. Cambridge, MA: Institute on Healthcare Improvement; 2014 [cited 10/14/2014]. Available from: http://www.ihi.org/education/ihiopenschool/Pages/default.aspx http://findit.library.jhu.edu/resolve?sid=Refworks%3AJohns%20Hopkins%20Institution&charset=utf-8&__char_set=utf8&genre=article&date=2014&atitle=IHI%20Open%20School&
13. Wachter RM, Pronovost PJ. Balancing "no blame" with accountability in patient safety. N Engl J Med. 2009;361:1401–6.
14. Pronovost PJ. Learning accountability for patient outcomes. JAMA. 2010;304(2):204–5.

House Staff Patient Safety Quality Council

Michelle Sharp

Tools
House Staff Patient Safety and Quality Council (HPSQC), Armstrong Institute for Patient Safety and Quality (AIPSQ), Accreditation Council for Graduate Medical Education (ACGME), project selection, "wow" factor, safety, financial impact, information technology (IT)

Summary of Council Structure

- The House Staff Patient Safety and Quality Council (HPSQC) functions as a council for quality and safety initiatives involving house staff members and reports to the Johns Hopkins Hospital Medical Board through the Patient Safety Committee and the Clinical Quality Improvement Committee. The major goals of the council are to:
  - Participate in the quality plan for the hospital by involving house staff in a meaningful way.

M. Sharp (✉)
Department of Pulmonary and Critical Care Medicine, John Hopkins University School of Medicine, Johns Hopkins Hospital, 1830 E. Monument Street, 5th floor, Baltimore, MD 21205, USA
e-mail: msharp5@jhmi.edu

L. Atanelov (ed.), *Resident's Handbook of Medical Quality and Safety*, DOI 10.1007/978-3-319-24190-6_8

- Partner with the Armstrong Institute for Patient Safety and Quality (AIPSQ), the Johns Hopkins Hospital Patient Safety Committee, the Johns Hopkins University Graduate Medical Education Committee, and the Johns Hopkins Hospital Medical Board to build capacity by training residents in patient safety and improvement methods.
- Serve as a unified voice for house staff as it relates to the organization's safety and quality improvement initiatives.
- Communicate key quality and patient safety information to the larger house staff community.
- Assist residency training programs in meeting the Accreditation Council for Graduate Medical Education (ACGME)-required education in "systems-based practice" and "practice-based learning and improvement" as core competencies.

- The counsel is made up of a senior and junior members from every residency throughout Johns Hopkins Hospital.
- The counsel has a faculty steering committee for counseling and guidance.
- Develop a yearly hospital-wide QI project. Past year examples include vaccine initiative and discharge project.
- Be the resident's voice on hospital patient safety committees.

Project Selection

- On a yearly basis, a project is selected.
- At the first meeting of the year, ideas are solicited from resident members.
- The steering committee meets to brainstorm ideas from the administration throughout the hospital.
- Individual projects are presented as possible ideas during the first two monthly meetings.
- Ideas are voted on by residents through an algorithm that assesses feasibility, multidisciplinary outcomes, "wow" factor, safety, and financial impact.

- Once a project is selected, the chair works on creating a project map with ideas and invites individuals throughout the hospital related to the project to meetings for discussion.
- An intervention is selected for the project and members are assigned with roles for assistance in the project:
  - Example: In the discharge project, it was realized from the brainstorm meeting and project map that the information technology (IT) department would be integral for the collection of data and intervention arm of the project. Our faculty advisors were able to suggest names of individuals to reach out to in IT. The chair coordinate a subcommittee to meet with several members of IT to discuss possible interventions through our data collection system. Once an intervention was selected, the coordinated with IT to arrange for data collection. Met with nursing leaders, physical and occupational and therapy leaders, case managers, and social workers to promote the project. The members of the council promoted the project within their respective residency programs. After the data was collected, the chair met with the administrative fellow and steering committee to discuss the analysis. The analysis was then presented to the council in the final meeting of the year.
- Once the project is completed, the data is presented to the medical board and hospital patient safety committee.
- The steering committee is able to supply advice for project ideas and guidance for implementation of the idea and overcoming challenges.

Successes

- Focus attention and discussions among residents about patient safety and quality.
- Collaboration of residents across the hospital joining in a united effort for improvement and change.
- Resident insight on various committees throughout the hospital.

- The HPSQC contributed in significant improvements in the hospital's vaccination rates for pneumococcal and influenza through collaboration with nursing and administration.
- The HPSQC investigated the discharge process throughout the JHH hospital and partnered with nursing, physical therapy/occupational therapy, case management, and social work on a communication project to help with the timeliness of discharge.
- The HPSQC has partnered with residency programs to choose/study a choosing wisely topic for each residency program.

Challenges

- Coordinating project across several different residencies.
- Finding time in resident's busy schedule to serve on HPSQC and providing dinner at meetings help with resident involvement/attendance.

If you have any questions about the information covered in this chapter or other medical safety and quality improvement-related topics, please contact us at http://www.medicalqualityandsafetyforum.com. The website will also provide a forum where you can ask specific questions about your safety and medical quality improvement projects or mentor upcoming medical quality leaders.

Part III
Sample QI Projects

Promoting Early Mobility for Hospitalized Patients: A Quality Improvement (QI) Project

DMAIC Phase: *Measure/Analyze*

Levi (Levan) Atanelov and Erik Hoyer

> **Tools**
> SBAR, DMAIC, Project-Y, PDCA, multivariable regression, survey, Project-X, Six Sigma, Lean, SMART goals, Johns Hopkins Highest Level of Mobility (JH-HLM)

Project Motivation (**SBAR***)

Situation (Practice Gap, the "Problem")

What

- Medical complications of bed rest in the hospital are well known.

L. Atanelov (✉)
Department of Physical Medicine and Rehabilitation, Johns Hopkins Hospital, Baltimore, MD, USA
e-mail: leviatanelov@gmail.com

E. Hoyer
Department of Physical Medicine and Rehabilitation, John Hopkins Hospital, Baltimore, MD, USA

L. Atanelov (ed.), *Resident's Handbook of Medical Quality and Safety*, DOI 10.1007/978-3-319-24190-6_9

- With proper training and the absence of contraindications, out-of-bed mobility and activity can be done safely and may be clinically beneficial to the patient.
- But, there often is a lack of:
  - Regular assessment of patient function during hospitalization
  - Interdisciplinary tools to communicate patient function
  - Prioritization to mobilize patients on a daily basis

How

- Observation from clinical experience

Background (Evidence, Context)

What

- Complications of bed rest are manifold and include venous thromboembolism, pressure ulcers, orthostatic hypotension, sinus tachycardia, hypercalcemia, atelectasis, aspiration pneumonia, constipation, and muscle weakness [should be referenced].
- Out-of-bed mobility and activity:
  - Can be performed safely
  - May reduce complications of bed rest (as above)
  - May reduce hospital length of stay even in the critically ill [1, 2]
- Patients spend a very large portion of their hospital stay lying in bed, and there is prevalent hospital culture that reinforces this [3].
- A large number of bed-rest orders are not medically indicated [4].
- Currently there is scarce documentation of patient functional status during the inpatient stay [5].

How

- PubMed searches
- Observation from clinical experience

Assessment (Conclusion)

- Despite the evidence, bed rest is common and may be associated with hospital-acquired harms.

Recommendations (Big Picture Plan of Action, "Project-Y")

- Training of providers.
- Algorithm for progressing patient mobility.
- Create an interface into the EMR to document patient impairment and the mobility that a patient actually performed during hospitalization.
- Discussion of patient function with multiproviders (i.e., care-coordination rounds).

Project Implementation (**DMAIC***)

Define

- Problem: Unnecessary bed rest commonly seen during the acute-care hospital can lead to functional impairment and increased medical complications.
- Goal: Create a transdisciplinary culture to promote mobility in hospitalized patients.
- Benefit: Reduce bed rest-associated medical complications.
- Scope: Two 24-bed general medicine units in a large teaching hospital.

Measure

What

- Identify perceived barriers to patient mobility.
- Measure patient mobility in the hospital.
- Measure length of stay during the QI project compared to 12 months prior to the intervention.

How

- We developed a survey to assess perceived barriers to patient mobility.
- We administered the survey to the medical care team (e.g., physicians, nurses, physical and occupational therapist) to identify baseline barriers to patient mobility.
- We develop a scale to measure patient mobility.
  - We created a metric called the Johns Hopkins Highest Level of Mobility (JH-HLM) (levels presented in Table 1).
- We worked closely with the information technology team to create an interface for documenting JH-HLM into the electronic medical records system and to automatically extract documented patient-mobility data.
- We engaged nursing staff to regularly document JH-HLM.
  - Educated nursing staff on importance of tracking patient mobility.
  - Measured compliance with JH-HLM documentation requirement (three times a day per patient).

Table 1 Johns Hopkins Highest Level of Mobility (JH-HLM) scale

		Score
Walk	250+ feet	8
	25+ feet	7
	10+ steps	6
Stand	≥1 min	5
Chair	Transfer to chair	4
Bed	Sit at edge of bed	3
	Turn self/bed activity[a]	2
	Only lying	1

[a]Bed activity includes passive or active range of motion, movement of arms or legs, bed exercises (e.g., cycle ergometry, neuromuscular electrical stimulation), and dependent transfer out of bed

– Kept nursing accountable for JH-HLM documentation.
– Provided regular feedback on JH-HLM documentation.
– Conducted weekly meetings to discuss challenges with JH-HLM documentation and propose solutions to these challenges.
– **PDCA*** cycle framework was utilized to *plan* ways to comply with JH-HLM documentation, *do* (execute) the discussed plans, *check* (evaluate) success of the plans, and *act* or identify corrective measures at regular meetings to improve compliance with JH-HLM documentation.

Analyze

What

- Analyze the survey results.
- Analyze compliance with JH-HLM documentation.
- Analyze barriers to JH-HLM documentation.

How

- Multivariable regression using R statistical software was used to identify variables associated with barriers to patient mobility (performed by attending).
- Run chart was used to display compliance with JH-HLM documentation.
- Conducted regular meetings with the nursing staff to discuss challenges with JH-HLM documentation (performed by attending).

Results

See Table 2.

Eighty two nurses and 32 physical and occupational therapists participated in the survey. Nurses perceived more barriers for mobility than PT/OTs. Perceived barriers to mobility

Table 2 Results of the survey

	Overall provider barriers scale	**Knowledge subscale**	**Attitudes subscale**	**Behaviors subscale**
	β (95 % CI)[a]	**β (95 % CI)[a]**	**β (95 % CI)[a]**	**β (95 % CI)[a]**
Experience (decades)	4 (1 to 7)*	5 (2 to 8)*	5 (1 to 8)	2 (−1 to 5)
RN	−32 (−39 to −26)*	−43 (−50 to −35)*	−21 (−28 to −14)*	−26 (−33 to −19)*
JHH	4 (−3 to11)	5 (−2 to 12)	3 (−4 to 9)	3 (−4 to 10)

*$p < 0.05$

[a]Multivariable linear regression models were used to examine the association of the Overall Provider Barriers Scale and subscales with the covariates described in the table. The results represent the difference in mean scale/subscale score (range of 0–100, with a lower score representing a higher barrier)

decreased with increased years of clinical practice. We also found that perceived barriers were similar between a large academic hospital compared with a community hospital, who also took the survey. Some of the specific barriers identified include lack of awareness of benefits of early ambulation of hospitalized patients, inertia of previous practice patterns, concerns about safety/time constraints, lack of skill toward identifying mobility needs, lack of motivation, and lack of staffing or training.

Compliance improved when team members were able to provide feedback to the unit nurse managers and bedside nurses their compliance data.

Improve

- See attending comments.

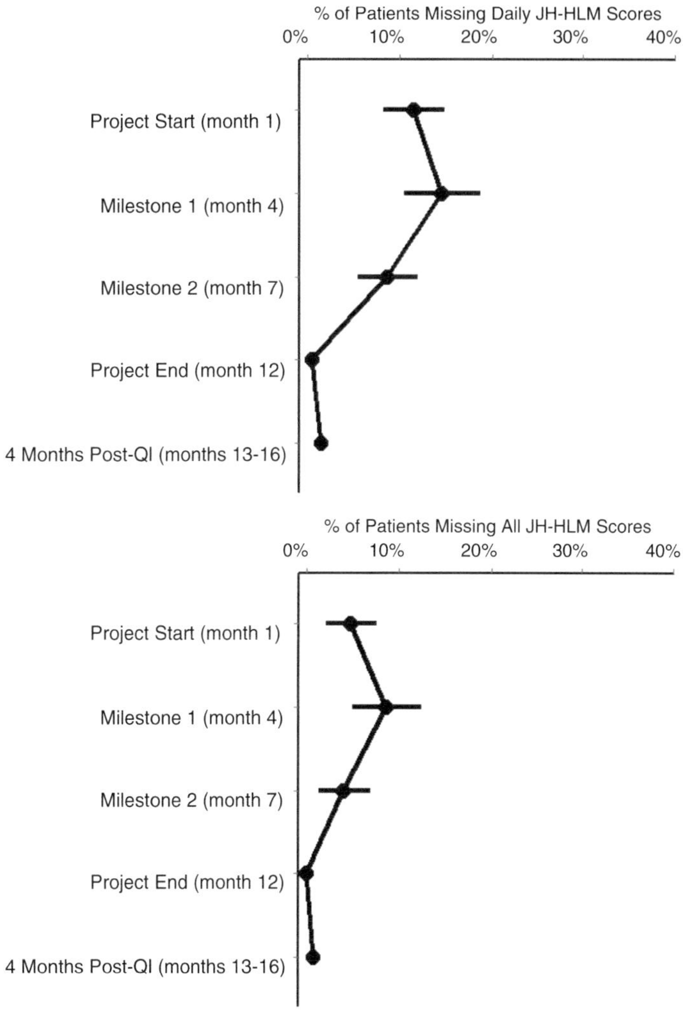

Fig. 1 Nursing adherence to documenting JH-HLM increases with time. Figure 1 generated by attending. Milestone 1 refers to when data was able to be extracted and reported back to the project units. Milestone 2 refers to nursing reeducation/engagement sessions. Error bars represent the 95 % confidence interval

Control

- See attending comments.

Challenges

- Scoping the project for resident schedule and goals.
- Setting a goal documentation-compliance rate using **SMART*** goals criteria prior to project implementation would have been helpful.
- Nursing compliance with JH-HLM documentation requirement was a challenge and required data-driven feedback to improve.

Successes

- With data feedback we were able to reach a high level of documentation compliance.

Attending Comments

- As an attending I utilized the resident by giving him focused components of the overall project including working on documents for the Institutional Review Board, working on documents to specify details for the data extraction, validation of the automated data extraction from the EMR, attending QI project team meetings, and developing questions on early drafts of the survey. The other aspects of the project included coordinating with managers, physicians, and administrative leaders and nurses to implement the project.
- As the attending I completed the analysis for the perceived barrier's survey and developed tools to calculate compliance rates and feedback reports using R statistical software.

- Since this was a pilot QI project and the JH-HLM scale was a novel scale for documenting patient function, it was built as an optional element in the EMR that nurses on those units had to specially add for their patients. It was critical for our QI team to provide nurse managers and champions feedback on nurse documentation compliance. We saw our greatest improvement in mobility scores (data not shown) and documentation compliance after the 4-month milestone when the automated data extract was completed, and we could provide the units with regular reports. Ultimately, we were able to work with nurses and administrators to pass a policy for functional assessment at Johns Hopkins Hospital, which incorporated the JH-HLM scale into standard nursing documentation workflows and resulted in sustainable (4 months post-QI project) documentation compliance.

Tools

SBAR

SBAR is a communication tool originally developed by the US Navy for use on nuclear submarines to enable consistent, succinct, accurate, and effective communication. SBAR was adopted into healthcare to reduce communication errors (e.g., nurse reporting a critical value to a physician) and promote patient safety. It has recently been shown to reduce incidents due to communication errors and improve patient safety culture [6].

- SBAR stands for situation, background, assessment, and recommendation.

Example

- Situation: Patient X has hemoglobin of 7.0.
- Background: Patient is post-op day 2; yesterday his hemoglobin was 9.0; he had been bleeding through his dressings.

- Assessment: Patient may be losing blood from his surgical wound.
- Recommendation: We should reassess his wound and consider blood transfusion.

DMAIC

DMAIC is a data-driven quality improvement framework often used with Six Sigma methodology developed to minimize waste in processes. The Six Sigma tool was originally developed by Motorola in the 1980s to reduce product variation. DMAIC provides a basic structure for Six Sigma implementation by providing a systematic approach to quality improvement projects. Six Sigma DMAIC tool was adapted to healthcare to guide quality improvement initiatives. For instance, DMAIC Six Sigma was used to streamline diagnosis of chest pain [7].

- DMAIC stands for define, measure, analyze, improve, and control.
- *Define* the problem at hand.
- *Measure* current baseline.
- *Analyze* and identify the specific causes of the problem.
- *Improve* and implement the intervention to reduce the problem.
- *Control* and ensure that the improvement phase lasts and ensure that deviations from goal performance are corrected without causing defects.

Example

- See different chapters in this book.
- Specific tools are available to facilitate each of these phases (see elsewhere).

PDCA Cycle

A systematic framework to foster a continuum of change developed by Walter Shewhart and made popular by Dr. Deming. PDCA was used in the manufacturing industry and had been adopted for healthcare needs [8]. The PDCA cycle churns continuously until desired results are accomplished and maintained.

- PDCA stands for plan, do, check, and act.
- *Plan*: An action plan or intervention is generated.
- *Do*: The intervention is executed.
- *Check:* The intervention is evaluated for success or failure.
- *Act:* Ideas generated to adjust the intervention to better approximate the desired outcome.

SMART Goals

SMART is a goal-setting technique to help develop goals that are easy to understand, execute, and evaluate (check that they have been accomplished). The SMART criteria are attributed to Peter Drucker. The term “SMART goals” is attributed to George T. Doran [9]. SMART goals have been used in healthcare, e.g., to assist with patient goal setting [10].

- SMART stands for specific, measurable, achievable, relevant, and time bound.
- Specific:
  - What: What do I want to accomplish?
  - Why: Specific reasons, purpose, or benefits of accomplishing the goal.
  - Who: Who is involved?
  - Where: Identify a location.
  - Which: Identify requirements and constraints.
- Measurable: Mathematically quantifiable outcome to mark level of goal attainment.
- Achievable: Realistic and attainable, clarify exactly how to achieve it.
- Relevant: Worthwhile, opportune (in time), apt for the team involved.
- Time-bound: Deadline helps focus team effort and allows for specific opportunity to evaluate accomplishment of the goal.

If you have any questions about the information covered in this chapter or other medical safety and quality improvement-related topics, please contact us at http://www.medicalqualityandsafetyforum.com. The website will also provide a forum where you can ask specific questions about your safety and medical quality improvement projects or mentor upcoming medical quality leaders.

References

1. Needham DM. Mobilizing patients in the intensive care unit: improving neuromuscular weakness and physical function. JAMA. 2008;300:1685–90.
2. Korupolu R, Gifford J, Needham DM. Early mobilization of critically ill patients: reducing neuromuscular complications after intensive care. Contemp Crit Care. 2009;6:1–12.
3. Brown CJ, Redden DT, Flood KL, Allman RM. The underrecognized epidemic of low mobility during hospitalization of older adults. J Am Geriatr Soc. 2009;57(9):1660–5.
4. Brown CJ, Friedkin RJ, Inouye SK. Prevalence and outcomes of low mobility in hospitalized older patients. J Am Geriatr Soc. 2004;52(8):1263–70.
5. Bogardus ST, et al. What does the medical record reveal about functional status? J Gen Intern Med. 2001;16:728–36.
6. Randmaa M, Mårtensson G, Leo Swenne C, Engström M. SBAR improves communication and safety climate and decreases incident reports due to communication errors in an anaesthetic clinic: a prospective intervention study. BMJ Open. 2014;4:e004268.
7. Kumar S, Thomas KM. Utilizing DMAIC six sigma and evidence-based medicine to streamline diagnosis in chest pain. Qual Manag Health Care. 2010;19:107–16.
8. Schroeder P. Using the PDCA cycle. Nurs Qual Connect. 1992;2:1–8.
9. Doran GT. There's a S.M.A.R.T. way to write management's goals and objectives. Manage Rev. 1981;70:35–6.
10. Bovend'Eerdt TJ, Botell RE, Wade DT. Writing SMART rehabilitation goals and achieving goal attainment scaling: a practical guide. Clin Rehabil. 2009;23:352–61.

Heart Sounds: Use of Audio Recordings to Improve Patient Discharge Communication

DMAIC Phase: *Define/Analyze*

Stacey L. Schott

Tools
DMAIC, Fishbone diagram, "Go to the Gemba", Survey, Value stream map, Voice of the customer, Voice of the Customer, Value Stream Mapping, Fishbone

Project Motivation (**SBAR***)

Situation (Practice Gap, the "Problem")

What

- Hospital reimbursement is tied to HCAHPS data and readmission rates.

S.L. Schott (✉)
Department of Internal Medicine, Johns Hopkins Bayview, 5200 Eastern Avenue, Mason F. Lord Building Center Tower, Baltimore, MD 21202, USA
e-mail: stacey.l.schott@hitchcock.org; schottlady@gmail.com

L. Atanelov (ed.), *Resident's Handbook of Medical Quality and Safety*, DOI 10.1007/978-3-319-24190-6_10

- Highest 30-day readmission rates at Johns Hopkins Bayview (JHB) tend to be in the progressive care unit (PCU) as of 7/31/13.

  Heart attack (22 %)
  Heart failure (29 %)
  Pneumonia (22 %)

- Despite the use of both *paper + verbal review* discharge process, patients in the JHB PCU report poor provider communication about medications and discharge instruction approximately 22 % of the time (CR).
- Correlates with communication/satisfaction scores in the 30th percentile or less statewide for this unit (JHB HCAHPS data Fall 2013).
- Ranks far below state mean on Press Ganey/HCAHPS.
- Poor communication is linked to increased readmission rates.

How

- Review of publicly reported data including Press Ganey/HCAHPS satisfaction scores, consumer reports based on data from the Centers for Medicare/Medicaid, and in-person patient surveys of patients

Background (Evidence, Context)

What

- Nearly 80 % of information doctors provide to patients verbally is immediately forgotten (within 1 min) [1].
- 50 % of information that *is* recalled is recalled incorrectly [2].
- Factors: age, health literacy, education, preferred learning style, and provider communication ability [3].
- Patients who understand their post-hospital care instructions are 30 % less likely to be readmitted [4].
- More than 50 % of patients across all health literacy levels preferred a modality of discharge instruction other than written or a combination of modalities [1].

How

- PubMed/Scopus/Google Scholar Search

Assessment (Conclusion)

- Effective provider–patient communication is critical for patients' ability to perform self-care after discharge.
- Standard *paper + verbal review* process of discharge instruction is failing to meet the complex communication needs of our patients.
- Communication failures appear to be impacting:
  - Readmission rates in complex, chronic conditions such as heart failure
  - Patients' ability to self-manage post-discharge care

Recommendations (Big Picture Plan of Action, "Project-Y")

- Provide a new, *free*, and reusable communication tool.
- Tool adds additional layer of communication to discharge process that better addresses discrepancies in health literacy and learning styles.
- Paper + verbal + *audio*.
- Replayable, virtually stored information (less likely to lose).
- Study and streamline discharge process to empower participation of discharging providers.

Project Implementation (**DMAIC***)

Define

- Problems
  - Cardiology unit inpatients are only moderately satisfied with the quality of provider communication about discharge instruction and report poor communication about new medications approximately 22 % of the time which contributes to decreased patient satisfaction

scores (30th percentile), decreased ability to self-manage care, increased 30-day readmission rates, and decreased hospital reimbursement rates.
  - Discharge communication patterns and styles are inconsistent; different providers (nurses/physicians).
  - Time to personalize communication to patient preference is limited.

- Goals
  - Change the discharge process to allow for higher quality, more personalized communication.
  - Improve patient understanding of medications and discharge instructions in order to enhance self-care after discharge (as measured by Discharge Knowledge Assessment Tool).
  - Improve patient satisfaction with provider discharge communication from moderately satisfied to extremely satisfied (as reported on post-hospital discharge surveys).
  - Increase HCAHPS communication scores from 30th percentile to consistently above 75th percentile.

- Benefits

  HARD: Decreased 30-day readmission rates in the cardiology PCU (heart failure patients), improved HCAHPS scores for discharge/medication communication, increased hospital reimbursement.

  SOFT: Increased ability to understand and execute self-care instructions, increased patient satisfaction

- Scope*:* Limited to cardiology service inpatients being discharged from PCU where resident physicians are always the primary discharging providers.

How

- Observe and document the current discharge process/work flow (Go to the Gemba).
- Survey of resident physician discharge instruction behaviors (VOC).

- Survey of patients' communication preferences (VOC).
- Survey of nursing discharge instruction behaviors (VOC).
- Value stream map of the current discharge process (VSM).

Tool

- **Go to the Gemba: A Japanese word for the "work area," or loosely "where the action is."** Go visit the work area: "Go see, ask why, show respect." Anyone can and should "Go to the Gemba." "It's amazing how well we think we know a process, but when we actually stand there and *watch* the process of work as it gets done, we see how different things are. We begin to see problems and opportunities for improvement and/or creativity." "Attempt to understand every gemba from the standpoints of *Purpose*, *Process* and *People*. Is management working to align people and process to achieve purpose? Are processes designed consistently to achieve the purpose? Are people engaged in working to achieve the purpose, and are they supported in this work by the processes?" **(From: www.lean.org).**
  – As applied to this project: Observed and participated in the discharge process of patients from the PCU. Documented patterns, behaviors, and physical work flows of providers. Considered how daily work flows could impact ability to provide consistently excellent and individualized communication. Recognized time constraints. Discussed and documented discharge communication preferences with patients.

Tool

- **Voice of the Customer (VOC):** A method used to capture the needs and wants of the customer (internal or external) as related to the process under investigation. VOC can be captured in a variety of ways: direct discussion or interviews, patient satisfaction surveys, focus groups, regulatory agency requirements, and observations. "If you don't improve your process based on customer needs/wants, your process improvement won't be successful." "What we assume our customers need/want may not be their actual needs and wants." Things constantly change in our customers' world. VOC helps you review what has changed in order to take the appropriate action **(From: Johns Hopkins Armstrong Institute for Patient Safety and Quality Prescription for Healthcare Lean Workshop).**

- As applied to this project: VOC surveys of patients in the cardiac PCU revealed deficiencies in the discharge communication system from the patient's perspective, identified a new modality through which they preferred to receive discharge information, and highlighted which care provider should be responsible to deliver this information to patients.

Tool

- **Value Stream Map:** "Let the map do the talking!" A visual depiction of "things" traveling through the various process steps (including materials and information) where waste and customer value can be identified. It includes *all* actions (of value and non-value) currently required to bring a product of service to the customer. It can identify "quick hits" for interventions. People commonly assume they know the process well without using VSM and fail to see the real and current state. Do not complete a value stream map without first observing the process! It requires going to the *Gemba* **(From: Johns Hopkins Armstrong Institute for Patient Safety and Quality Prescription for Healthcare Lean Workshop**).
- As applied to this project:
- Helped to identify inconsistency/redundancy in the discharge process (only nurse performing discharge vs. only physician performing discharge vs. both nurse and physician duplicating discharge at separate times, providing inconsistent and potentially confusing information).
- Helped to identify areas of inefficiency/delay. See Fig. 1.

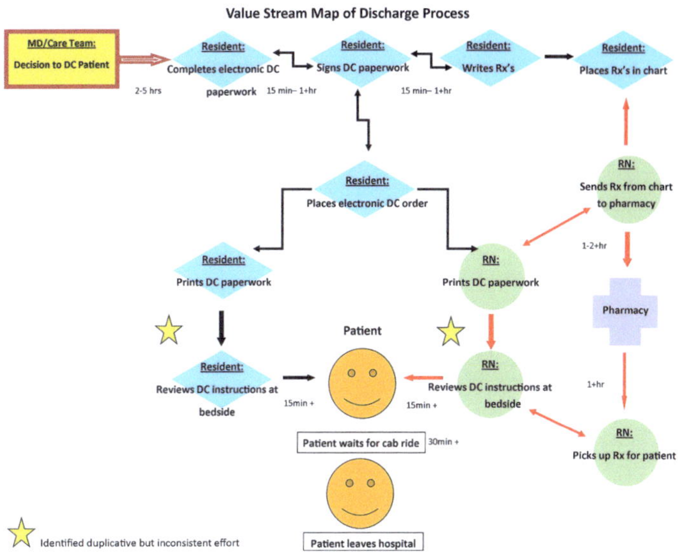

FIG. 1 Value Stream Map of patient discharge process

Measure: Pre-Pilot (See results)

What

Patient:

- Perception of/satisfaction with current discharge process
- Preference for who communicates instructions (nurse vs. physician)
- Preferred modality of discharge instruction (audio vs. traditional)

Physician:

- Perception of current discharge process
- Preference for who communicates instructions (nurse vs. physician)
- Preferred modality of discharge instruction (audio vs. traditional)

Nurse:

- Perception of current discharge process
- Preference for who communicates instructions (nurse vs. physician)
- Preferred modality of discharge instruction (audio vs. traditional)

How: Survey

Results of the pre-pilot surveys

Patients: ($n = 12$)
- Only moderately satisfied with current discharge process
- Frequently lose paper
- 92 % prefer physician to communicate discharge instruction
- 92 % prefer audio recording vs. traditional instruction
- 100 % would share audio with caretakers or family
- Plan to replay until learned
- 66 % had access to email ± smartphone
- Barrier: access to technology decreases with age (range: 39–87)

Resident physicians: ($n = 40$)
- 93 % believe they should be responsible for discharge instruction
- But only 60 % reported *they* usually verbally review instructions
- Estimated that nurses reviewed instructions 28 % of the time
- 5 % felt physicians + nurses should review instructions
- 87.9 % felt comfortable having their discharge conversation recorded
- Barrier: time

Nurses: ($n = 16$)
- Wide variation in percentage of nurses who report completing discharge task routinely
- Nurses with more experience were more likely to *always* verbally review discharge instructions
- 100 % preferred physician + nurse completed discharge
- Approximately 50 % felt comfortable having their discharge conversation recorded
- Barrier: unsure about details of care

Patients identified they were only moderately satisfied with the current process of communication at discharge and generally preferred that physicians communicate with them at the point of discharge. Resident physician perceptions of responsibility for discharge varied from their actual performance of discharge communication. They identified time as the biggest barrier to consistent and effective discharge communication. Nurses confirmed the variability in which physician providers actually performed the discharge communication. 100 % preferred the physician completes this task, but most often more experienced nurses took ownership of completing the discharge communication encounter. The majority of patients, resident physicians, and nurses were open to participating in an audio recording of the discharge communication process. (Data were altered for the purposes of demonstration, but remain consistent with ongoing study findings thus far).

Analyze

What

- Analyze the current discharge process.
- Analyze barriers to discharge communication.

How

- Fishbone diagram of factors contributing to poor communication.

Tool

- **Fishbone diagram**; "Cause and effect" diagram. A graphical method used in conjunction with brainstorming to identify, logically group, and subdivide potential root causes of a problem. Spine of the fish is the problem or key metric. The "fins" are the 6 M's – man (personnel), machines, material, methods, measurements, and mother nature (environment). Can help you pinpoint an area

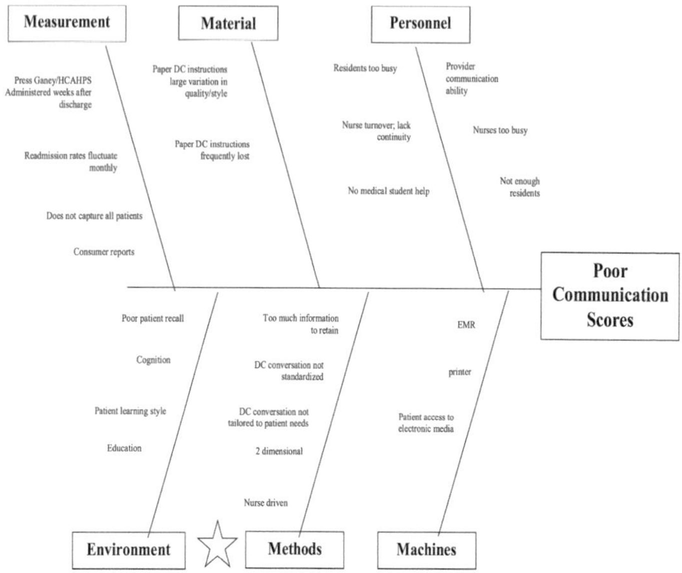

FIG. 2 Fishbone Diagram used as part of a Root Cause Analysis of poor communication scores

upon which to intervene **(From: Johns Hopkins Armstrong Institute for Patient Safety and Quality Prescription for Healthcare Lean Workshop).**

- As applied to this project:
- The fishbone tool identified that the *methods* being used to discharge a patient may be impacting effective communication; the identified *method* was within the control of the provider and therefore chosen as a viable target for change. See Fig. 2.

Improve: Audio intervention devised as a result of completing the DMAIC improvement process.

- Patients with smartphone, email, or recordable device will be randomized to:
- Group 1: (paper + verbal instructions)
- Group 2: (paper + verbal + audio instructions)

- All discharge communications recorded to minimize Hawthorne effect and then randomized to group 1 or group 2.
- Both groups contacted by phone 2 weeks after discharge to complete communication survey + Discharge Knowledge Assessment.
- Satisfaction scores from communication survey and Discharge Knowledge Assessment scores compared between groups 1 and 2 to determine the impact of audio instruction on satisfaction and understanding of self-managed care.

Control: Post-Pilot

- Long-term goal: To compare HCAHPS scores pre- and post-pilot study to determine whether or not satisfaction scores increase (and can be tied to intervention).
- Ensure easy access to recording system for next generation of discharging providers.

If proves successful:

- May serve to help standardize discharge process; expectation that physician routinely responsible for discharge communication *at* bedside
- May serve as educational tool for discharging provider to review, analyze, and improve upon quality of verbal discharge behaviors/bedside information delivery.
- May provide evidence for investment in other devices/platforms where patients can routinely access (*embed audio recording into Epic MyChart (EMR) for easier patient and colleague access*)

Challenges

- Never bring personal presumptions to the table; be a blank slate, *observe*, *learn*, and then analyze and come up with a plan *based* solely on the defined problem *as the "customer" perceives it*. Do not bring *ideas* first; base ideas on actual problems; clearly define problems first.

- Change intervention to design more like a "study" that is valid and publishable; search for "evidence" that audio recordings impact patient's understanding of self-care → more powerful message in quality improvement.
- IRB applications may delay project unexpectedly; attempt to work on other aspects while waiting.
- Maintaining team interest and participation along the way.

Successes

- Developed and maintained leadership aspect over pilot project
- Gained significant education in elements required for design and approval of project/study through IRB
- Learned how to effectively partner with hospital leadership and cardiology unit colleagues to promote quality care
- Increased passion for career in improving quality in healthcare communication

If you have any questions about the information covered in this chapter or other medical safety and quality improvement-related topics, please contact us at http://www.medicalqualityandsafetyforum.com. The website will also provide a forum where you can ask specific questions about your safety and medical quality improvement projects or mentor upcoming medical quality leaders.

References

1. Chugh, A, Williams, M et al. Betters Transitions: Improving Comprehension of Discharge Instructions. Frontiers in Health Services Management. 2009;25:3.
2. Olives,T. Paper ED instructions: Ready, set, delete. Annual Meeting for the Society of Academic Emergency Medicine. 2012. http://www.emed-journal.com/articles/practice-economics-news/article/paper-ed-discharge-instructions-ready-set-delete/3794efe78d21c4d8c6a6de6f8b2f2b10.html.

3. Kessels, R. Patients' memory for medical information. J R Soc Med. 2003; 96(5):219–222.
4. Bailey, C. Nursing Management: Reducing readmissions through discharge communication. Nursing Management. http://journals.lww.com/nursingmanagement/toc/2012/12001. 2012; 43(12):14–16.
5. Johns Hopkins Bayview HCAHPS data (July 2013-Fall 2013).

Smoking Cessation in Pregnancy and Beyond: A Quality Improvement (QI) Project

DMAIC Phase: *Define*

Marielle S. Gross

> **Tools**
> Define, Measure, Analyze, Improve, and Control (DMAIC) and Situation, Background, Assessment, Recommendation (SBAR)

Situation: ***Define*** *the Problem*

- Medical complications of smoking during pregnancy are well known [1, 2].
- Women are motivated to quit during pregnancy and are often successful [1–4].

Project Motivation: Situation, Background, Assessment, Recommendation (SBAR) and Define, Measure, Analyze, Improve, and Control (DMAIC) tools

M.S. Gross (✉)
Department of Gynecology and Obstetrics, John Hopkins University School of Medicine, 600 Wolfe Street, Phipps #279, Baltimore, MD 21287, USA
e-mail: mgross23@jhmi.edu

L. Atanelov (ed.), *Resident's Handbook of Medical Quality and Safety*, DOI 10.1007/978-3-319-24190-6_11

- Brief provider interventions are effective for promoting and maintaining cessation [2–5].
- Little anticipatory guidance is provided and postpartum recidivism is high [6].

How

- Clinical observation, American College of Obstetricians and Gynecologists (ACOG) recommendations, and PubMed searches

Background: ***Measure*** *the Harms of Smoking in Pregnancy*

- Smoking causes abnormal placentation, intrauterine growth restriction, and premature delivery [2].
- Smoking increases perinatal mortality and ectopic pregnancy rates [2].
- Children have increased risk of respiratory infections, asthma, infantile colic, sudden infant death syndrome (SIDS), middle ear disease, atherogenesis, childhood obesity, and behavioral problems [2].
- 23 % of American women report smoking in the 3 months before pregnancy [2, 7].
- 46 % of prepregnancy smokers quit directly before or during pregnancy [2, 4, 5, 7].
- Up to 60 % of those who quit during pregnancy return to smoking within 1 year postpartum [2, 4, 7].
- The American Academy of Pediatrics (AAP) prescribes eight well-child visits in the first year of life.
- There is no protocol for ensuring continuity of care between obstetricians and pediatricians with respect to the mutually imperative goal of maternal smoking cessation and abstinence [4, 5].

How

- Clinical observation, ACOG data, AAP Bright Futures Guidelines, and PubMed searches

*Assessment: **Analyze** the Potential for Quality Improvement*

- Promoting smoking cessation intra- and postpartum is a vital, well-defined public health goal [2].
- Women successfully quit in pregnancy, but postpartum recidivism is unacceptably high [2, 4, 5, 7].
- Anticipatory guidance is not emphasized, and there are missed opportunities to provide continuity of care for smoking cessation and abstinence [6].
- Quality of care is compromised by a deficiency in interdisciplinary communication.

*Recommendations: How Can We **Improve** the Quality of Smoking Cessation Care in This Population?*

- Promote interdisciplinary coordination to improve quality and continuity of care for smoking cessation and abstinence with *enhanced force functionality in EPIC electronic medical records.*
- Encourage *obstetricians* to provide ongoing smoking cessation and anticipatory guidance to prevent smoking relapse during the routine obstetric visits:
  - Prompt physicians to provide at least one of the cost-effective ACOG and Cochrane Review-endorsed interventions, such as "Motivational Interviewing" [2, 3, 5].
  - Create a "hard stop" to closing an outpatient encounter for patients with smoking history, asking about staging of patient within the transtheoretical model: precontemplation, contemplation, preparation, action, or maintenance, which interventions were provided postpartum plans for abstinence and barriers to cessation [4, 5].
  - Work with EPIC IT staff to modify existing templates; provide physicians, nurses, and social workers with training, resources, and aids for incorporating quick, effective counseling into their patient encounters.

- Engaging *pediatricians* starts when anticipated pediatric care site is identified as per the routine obstetric standard of care checklist:
  - Seek support from pediatrics colleagues, including NICU faculty and staff, residents, and specifically those who have experience with smoking cessation research and/or pediatric complications of maternal smoking.
  - Pediatricians can provide ongoing support to prevent relapse utilizing the electronic medical record; we will provide them with similar training and resources for reinforcing anti-smoking messages [3–5].
  - We will modify existing well-child exam templates to automatically import relevant data from aforementioned routine obstetric visits.
  - Sample auto-populated questions: Is there 'in utero' tobacco exposure to cigarette smoke? Are there smoking-related pregnancy or neonatal complications? Did mother quit during pregnancy? Stages of change: Where is she now? Are there other smokers in the home? We will work with IT to create a similar "hard stop" for the well-child encounter [3–5].

Methods

- Inclusion criteria: resident and high-risk obstetric clinic patients and current smokers or those who quit immediately before or during pregnancy, presenting for routine obstetric care
- Enrollment goal: 500 patients
- Randomization: 100 patients control group, 400 patients in treatment group
- Frequency of routine obstetric and pediatric visits: same as current standard of care
- Length of study: 3 years, with enrollment of patients for first 15 months and final follow-up assessment at 1-year well-child visit; data for controls can begin being collected right away
- Sites involved: Johns Hopkins Hospital and Johns Hopkins Bayview Obstetrics and Pediatrics clinics

End Points

- Gather data on *prevalence of smoking* upon admission for delivery and at 1-month, 6-month, and 1-year well-child visits.
- We will also gather data on premature birthrate and smoking-associated pregnancy complications as well as pediatric URI diagnoses, asthma diagnoses, and hospitalizations.

Future Plans

- Analysis of smoking rates with a *t*-test at the conclusion of the 3-year study will determine if this model is an improvement over the current standard of care.
- Close the loop by importing data from pediatric patient records into mother's chart for subsequent pregnancies.

Challenges to Address Prior to Implementation

- Determine if this model is problematic for pediatricians regarding insurance and reimbursement for providing services to their patients indirectly by counseling their mothers.
- Our hospital system is currently transitioning from QS to EPIC for outpatient obstetric care.
- This project requires a multidisciplinary approach, with obstetricians, pediatricians, affiliated nurse providers, and EPIC IT.

Limitations

- This only works for patients who receive both obstetric and pediatric care under the JHMI system.

- Study sample size will likely be underpowered to detect a clinically significant difference in rates of some important but relatively rare outcomes, such as SIDS.
- This intervention could potentially lengthen the visit time and burden time-pressed providers.

Conclusion

- Despite its limitations, the implementation of a force-function-enriched smoking cessation program is straightforward and feasible and presents no greater risk over current standard of care. The cost-to-benefit ratio is favorable and potential gains exceed the effort and expense in initiating this program.
- If successful, this model lends itself to expansion to other relevant health issues.

If you have any questions about the information covered in this chapter or other medical safety and quality improvement-related topics, please contact us at http://www.medicalqualityandsafetyforum.com. The website will also provide a forum where you can ask specific questions about your safety and medical quality improvement projects or mentor upcoming medical quality leaders.

References

1. Dietz PM, England LJ, Shapiro-Mendoza CK, Tong VT, Farr SL, Callaghan WM. Infant morbidity and mortality attributable to prenatal smoking in the US. Am J Prev Med. 2010;39:45–52.
2. Smoking cessation during pregnancy. Committee Opinion No. 471. American College of Obstetricians and Gynecologists. Obstet Gynecol 2010;116:1241–4.
3. Chamberlain C, O'Mara-Eves A, Oliver S, et al. Psychosocial interventions for supporting women to stop smoking in pregnancy. Cochrane Database Syst Rev. 2013;10:CD001055.

4. Pletsch PK. A model for postpartum smoking resumption prevention for women who stop smoking while pregnant. J Obstet Gynecol Neonatal Nurs. 2006;35:215–22.
5. Valanis B, et al. Maternal smoking cessation and relapse prevention during health care visits. Am J Prev Med. 2001;20(1):1–8.
6. Zapka JG, Pbert L, Stoddard AM, Ockene JK, Goins KV, Bonollo D. Smoking cessation counseling with pregnant and postpartum women: a survey of community health center providers. Am J Public Health. 2000;90:78–84.
7. Colman GJ, Joyce T. Trends in smoking before, during, and after pregnancy in ten states. Am J Prev Med. 2003;24:29–35.

Facilitating Early-In-Day Discharge for Multiple Sclerosis Patients Treated with Intravenous Methylprednisolone: A Quality Improvement (QI) Project

DMAIC Phase: *Control*

John C. Probasco

> **Tools**
> Checklist, DMAIC, Lean Six Sigma Process Map, Order set, and SBAR

J.C. Probasco, MD (✉)
Department of Neurology, Johns Hopkins Hospital,
600 North Wolfe Street, Meyer 6-113, Baltimore, MD 21287, USA
e-mail: jprobas1@jhmi.edu

L. Atanelov (ed.), *Resident's Handbook of Medical Quality and Safety*, DOI 10.1007/978-3-319-24190-6_12

Project Motivation (**SBAR***)

Situation (Practice Gap, the "Problem")

What

- Delays in patient discharges from the hospital can have upstream effects on patient movement within the hospital.
- Coordinating care and planning for discharge from the time of admission and throughout the course of hospitalization can facilitate early-in-day discharge.
- Care can be poorly coordinated between members of the care team (e.g., nursing staff, therapists, social workers, house staff, attending physicians).
- Discharge preparations are often not begun from time of admission and/or well communicated between members of the care team and with patients.

How

- Observation from clinical experience

Background (Evidence, Context)

What

- Delays in patient discharges from the hospital can have upstream effects on patient movement within the hospital, such as from critical care units and the emergency department [1].
- Persistent delays in patient discharges can culminate in the cancellation of direct admissions and scheduled procedures as well as the inability to admit patients from the emergency department [2, 3].
- Delays in patient discharges lead to increased length of stay, diminished patient satisfaction in care, and diminished hospital staff satisfaction [4].
- Early-in-day patient discharges have been described as a means of alleviating hospital patient flow bottlenecks [5].

- Early-in-day discharge of patients is an achievable and sustainable goal, well demonstrated in the general medicine inpatient population [6, 7].
- Early-in-day discharge has previously been facilitated by practices including [6, 7]:
    - Estimating a patient's anticipated length of stay
    - Communication of this estimate to patients
    - Communication of this estimate to other care team members
    - Continued assessment of barriers to discharge throughout the course of hospitalization
    - Dividing tasks necessary for safe discharge and outpatient transition among members of the care team
    - Engaging patients in discharge preparations
    - Completing tasks for discharge prior to day of discharge, as able (e.g., discharge paperwork, scheduling appointments, coordinating services)
    - Utilizing checklists for activities of safe discharge planning

How

- Observation and clinical experience of multiple members of the care team

Assessment (Conclusion)

- Poor coordination throughout the course of hospitalization and in the discharge process leads to delays in discharge.
- Preparations for discharge are often not begun until day of discharge.

Recommendations (Big Picture Plan of Action, "Project-Y")

- Prepare for day of discharge from time of admission, *in order to*
- Facilitate early-in-day discharge

Project Implementation (**DMAIC***)

Define

- Problem: Poor coordination of care and discharge preparation lead to low frequency of early-in-day discharge.
- Goal: Increase frequency of early-in-day discharge of patients admitted for acute exacerbation of multiple sclerosis and treated with intravenous steroids.
- Benefit: Improve patient flow by reducing discharge bottleneck.
- Scope: Two medical-surgical nursing units.

Measure

What

- Describe course of hospitalization and discharge process for patients with multiple sclerosis admitted for acute exacerbations and treatment with intravenous steroids.
- Measure baseline time intervals for points of care and interventions throughout hospitalization as well as discharge process.
- Measure baseline rate of early-in-day discharge.

How

- Develop a process map of hospitalization and discharge for candidate patient population. Identify areas of delay and opportunities for better care coordination. (*Lean Six Sigma Process Map**, Fig. 1)
- Discuss the process map and identify areas of delay and opportunities for better care coordination with all members of the care team.
- From this process map, develop an intervention to better coordinate providers.
    - We created an intervention order set within the electronic medical record system which facilitated the scheduling of timed doses of steroids on an advancing

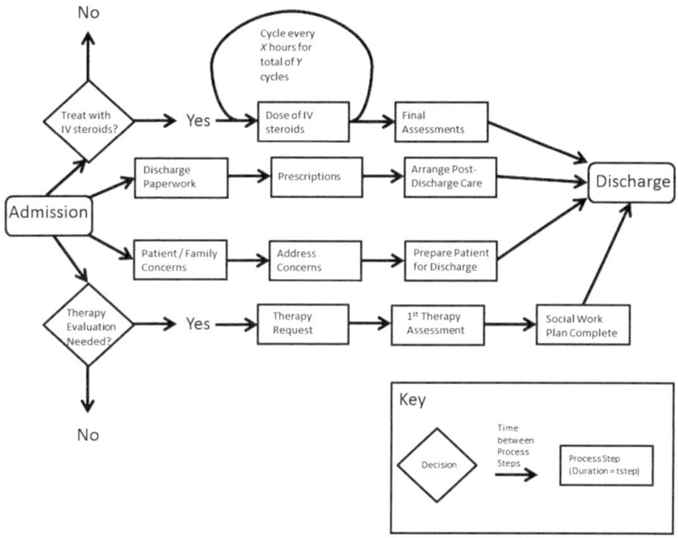

FIG. 1 Simplified process map for facilitating early-in-day discharge for multiple sclerosis patients treated with intravenous methylprednisolone. This figure is now in publication: Neurohospitalist. 2015 Oct;5(4):197-204. doi: 10.1177/1941874415576206.

schedule to allow for early-in-day administration of the final dose on the last planned day of admission.
- We included order options for needed diagnostic testing.
- We instructed nursing staff to distribute a patient checklist for admission (discussed below) and information on the use of intravenous steroids in acute exacerbations of multiple sclerosis.

- We created a provider checklist that was entered in the electronic handoff available for review and use by all members of the care team. It included:
  - Date of admission
  - Anticipated date of discharge
  - Time of first steroid dose
  - Scheduled time of final steroid dose
  - Tasks to be completed to facilitate early-in-day discharge, including:

    - Request and completion of therapy assessments as appropriate
    - Discussion of patient transportation home on day of discharge
    - Writing and filling of prescriptions
    - Completion of discharge paperwork

- We created a patient checklist which included:
    - Date of anticipated discharge
    - Tasks to be completed during hospitalization (e.g., imaging studies, therapy assessments)
    - Coordination of transportation home
    - Receipt of needed prescriptions
    - Review of home medications and any medication changes
    - Answering of all questions regarding hospitalization
    - Arrangement of follow-up appointments

Analyze

What

- Analyze utilization of intervention order set (with instruction for distribution of patient checklist and education sheet) and provider checklist.
- Analyze barriers to order set utilization, provider checklist utilization, and distribution of patient materials.
- Analyze metrics of care coordination, discharge coordination, and frequency of early-in-day discharge and compare to a retrospective baseline sample.

How

- Conduct regular meetings of multidisciplinary project team to analyze barriers to provider checklist utilization, patient checklist distribution, and patient education sheet distribution.

- Conduct regular meetings with house staff and general neurology inpatient providers regarding utilization of provider order set and provider checklist.
- Evaluate the following with comparison to a retrospective baseline sample by nonparametric tests, as appropriate:
  - Frequency of early-in-day discharge
  - Frequency of early-in-day final treatment
  - Frequency of discharge on same day as final treatment
  - Time from request for therapy assessment and assessment by therapist
  - Time from last infusion of intravenous steroids and discharge
  - Length of stay
  - 30-day readmission rate

Results (Note: Original Data Was Altered for Purposes of Reporting in This Book)

After a period of developing the interventions and provider training on utilization of the intervention order set and provider checklist, providers achieved a rate of 80 % utilization of either intervention.

The hospital admissions and discharge process were evaluated prospectively for 26 consecutive intervention patients and were compared to a retrospective sample of 24 consecutive patients that was well matched in terms of age, gender, and morbidity.

In the intervention period, there was a threefold increase in the frequency of early-in-day discharge (Fig. 2). This was in the setting of a similar increase in the rate of early-in-day completion of treatment. There was also a trend toward more patients being discharged on the same day as their final treatment. There was no change in the time intervals from request for therapy assessment and assessment and from final treatment to discharge. Of note, there was no change in the rate of 30-day readmissions, a gross measure of care quality.

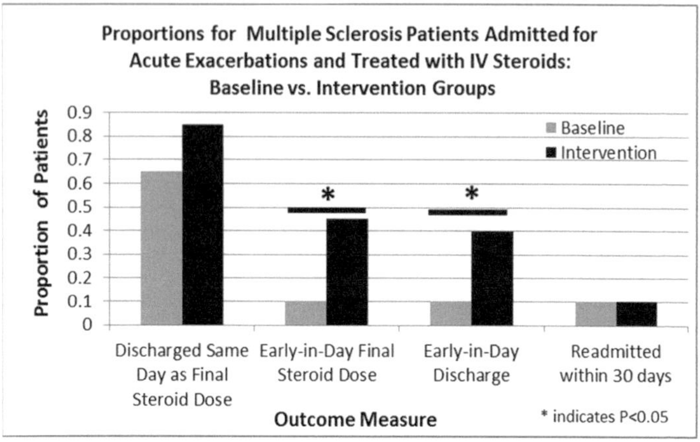

FIG. 2 Intervention led to increase in frequency of early-in-day completion of treatment and discharge without affecting care quality (Note: Original data was altered for purposes of reporting in this book)

Control

Currently monitoring for sustained frequency of intervention utilization and rate of early-in-day discharge. Also, a manuscript detailing this project and results is being prepared for publication.

Challenges

- Developing intervention order set and process for formal review and approval at the hospital level
- Troubleshooting barriers to utilization of intervention order set and utilization of provider checklist by house staff
- Accounting for influence of concurrent departmental and care unit efforts which may confound results
- Formal assessment of patient utilization of checklist, survey regarding patient checklist, and provided information yet to be performed

Successes

- Learning by experience
- Proof of concept of care coordination from time of admission in facilitating early-in-day discharge

Tools

Lean Six Sigma Process Map (Fig. 1)

Lean Six Sigma is a managerial concept centered on the elimination of various forms of waste (referred to as *muda*) from processes. Types of *muda* include defects, waiting, non-utilized talent, overproduction, transportation, inventory, unnecessary movement, and over-processing. A process map is a visual document which presents a process. It includes data related to the process such as steps in the process, time associated with completions of each step, and time between steps. It provides a description of a process to help understand problems associated with the process, allowing teams to easily recognize improvement opportunities within the process and underlying causes of such problems. It also helps teams to visualize how the process should work. Finally, it is a useful communication tool for presentation to others within and outside the project team [8].

If you have any questions about the information covered in this chapter or other medical safety and quality improvement-related topics, please contact us at http://www.medicalqualityandsafetyforum.com. The website will also provide a forum where you can ask specific questions about your safety and medical quality improvement projects or mentor upcoming medical quality leaders.

Acknowledgments The chapter author would like to acknowledge the contributions of the following team members to the project presented here: Gina Hawley, DrPH; Margie Burnett, RN BSN CNRN; Lorrie Gibson, MSIT; Kathryn Carter, MS PA-C; Elizabeth Harlow, RN BSN CNRN; Holly Russell, MS OTR/L; Linda Huffman, RN MSN; Jane Adams, RN BSN CNRN; Terry Ziegler, MSW; Hilary Sporney, RN SCM MBA; Michael Levy, MD, PhD; and Hans A. Puttgen, MD. The author would also like to acknowledge the efforts of the neurosciences acute care unit staff as well as the neurology faculty and house staff who participated in this quality improvement project.

References

1. Proudlove NC, Boaden R. Using operational information and information systems to improve in-patient flow in hospitals. J Health Organ Manage. 2005;19:466–77.
2. Rich V, Sullivan P, Kirby A. Pioneers in patient flow improvement: combining people, processes, and technology. Nurs Leader. 2007;5:52–6.
3. Jweinat J, Damore P, Morris V, D'Aquila R, Bacon S, Balcezak TJ. The safe patient flow initiative: a collaborative quality improvement journey at Yale-New Haven Hospital. Jt Comm J Qual Patient Saf. 2013;39(10):447–59.
4. Khanna S, Boyle J, Good N, Lind J. Impact of admission and discharge peak times on hospital overcrowding. Stud Health Technol Inform. 2011;168:82–8.
5. Derlat RW, Richards JR. Overcrowding in the nation's emergency departments: complex causes and disturbing effects. Ann Emerg Med. 2000;35(1):63–8.
6. Kravett SJ, Levine RB, Rubin HR, Wright SM. Discharging patients earlier in the day: a concept worth evaluating. Health Care Manage. 2007;26(2):142–6.
7. Wertheimer B, Jacobs REA, Bailey M, Holstein S, Chatfield S, Ohta B, Horrocks A, Hockman K. Discharge before noon: an achievable hospital goal. J Hosp Med. 2014;9(4):210–4.
8. George ML, Rowlands D, Price M, Maxey J. Process mapping. In: The lean six sigma pocket toolbook. New York: McGraw Hill; 2005. pp. 34–46.

Improving Compliance with Vaccination Core Measures

DMAIC Phase: *Control*

Susan Peterson and Brent Petty

> **Tools**
>
> Cause and effect matrix, SBAR, DMAIC, House Staff Patient Safety and Quality Council (HPSQC), "wow"factor, patient effect, outcomes, feasibility, multi-disciplinary nature

S. Peterson (✉)
Department of Emergency Medicine, Johns Hopkins University School of Medicine, 1830 E. Monument Street, Suite 6-100, Baltimore, MD 21287, USA
e-mail: speter14@jhmi.edu

B. Petty
Department of Medicine, John Hopkins Hospital, Baltimore, MD, USA

L. Atanelov (ed.), *Resident's Handbook of Medical Quality and Safety*, DOI 10.1007/978-3-319-24190-6_13

Project Motivation (SBAR)

Situation

What

- Compliance for the "global immunization" core measure for influenza and pneumococcal pneumonia was significantly below the institutional goals of >96 % compliance in 2012.
- A comprehensive order set was created by the institution; however, compliance rates continued to be well below the goal of greater than 96 % [1].

How

- Compliance rates were collected, compiled, and recorded by the central hospital based on core measure methodology.

Background

What

- Global immunization for influenza and pneumococcal pneumonia became a core measure in January 2012.
- The institution chose to adhere strictly to CDC guidelines for these vaccinations in order to avoid over-vaccination [2].
    - While guidelines for administration of influenza vaccination were relatively straightforward, guidelines for administration of pneumococcal vaccination were more complex and were often found to be a source of inappropriate ordering practices.
- The Housestaff Patient Safety and Quality Council (HPSQC) was created in the summer of 2012 with a vision to create house staff-driven improvement of patient care and involve house staff in the existing quality improvement structure.
- In its inaugural year, the HPSQC wanted to choose a QI project in order to meet its goals. A cause and effect matrix (Fig. 1) was used to determine which project would have the greatest impact and where we should direct our efforts.

CAUSE & EFFECT MATRIX

Importance of Customers	1	1	1	1	1	1	1						
Customer Rank													
KPIV / KPOV	feasibility	Mulit disciplinar y	outcomes	Wow factor	safety	Financial impact	patient effect				Rank	Rating	Total
Blood prod Utilization													0.00
Choosing Wisely													0.00
ED/Hostpital flow													0.00
Cardiac Enzymes													0.00
Vaccination Project													0.00

FIG. I Cause and effect matrix

- Effects that we were seeking included safety, outcomes, "wow" factor, feasibility, patient effect, and multidisciplinary nature.
  - Each effect was given a rank of importance (listed as "customer rank" on the example matrix below) from one to ten.
- Each cause, or potential project in this case, was given a value that related to how much of an effect it would have for the respective category.
  - For example, the vaccination project was considered to be very feasible and was given a score of eight in that cell.
- The "customer rank" of the effect was then multiplied by the value assigned to the effect. These values were added to give the project a rating and the highest rating project was given the highest rank.

– The HPSQC chose improving compliance with "global immunizations" as an interdisciplinary quality improvement project based on the results of the cause and effect matrix exercise.

– When the Council initiated its project by discussing vaccination screening with members of the hospital's QI team, the following was revealed:

- HPSQC members did not know why the existing vaccination order set had been put in place

- HPSQC members were not aware of the core measure for immunization or the hospital's compliance rate on this measure.
- HPSQC members were not familiar with the specifics of the CDC vaccination guidelines
- While a concurrent review process existed, when this was discussed with the HPSQC it was clear that the concurrent reviewers did not have a clear idea of whom to contact to order vaccination screening that had not been ordered correctly per the existing order set.

How

- Compliance rates were already collected, compiled, and recorded by the hospital based on core measure methodology, and this practice continued through the implementation of the project.
- The HPSQC met monthly. The HPSQC leadership had an additional monthly meeting in order to direct the goals of the project. The HPSQC leadership also met monthly with the institutional quality improvement vaccination team.

Assessment

- Compliance rates were below goal because the purpose of the order set was poorly understood, there was little knowledge about the "global immunization core measures" by house staff who ordered the majority of these vaccinations, and communication regarding immunization failures was poorly understood.

Recommendations

- Implementation of an education slide set created by house staff about the core measure and distributed by HPSQC members to their respective departmental house staff colleagues
- Creation of a competition between departments for most compliant and most improved department

– Partnering with the quality improvement staff in order to optimize the concurrent review process and communication plan for inadequate screening for vaccination

Project Implementation: DMAIC

Define

Problem: Compliance with "global immunizations" for influenza and pneumococcal pneumonia.
Goal: Improvement of compliance to >96 %.
Benefit: Decrease the potential for future morbidity of inpatients.
Scope: Inpatients of the Johns Hopkins Hospital.

Measure

What

Compliance rates for pneumococcal pneumonia vaccinations and influenza vaccinations by department.
Failure to order the vaccination correctly was also tracked and reviewed by the concurrent review team in conjunction with leadership of the HPSQC.

How

– CMS vaccination core measure methodology [3]:

  - 104 medical record numbers of admitted patients were randomly selected and reviewed by the QI staff to determine compliance.
  - From those 104 medical record numbers, patients who were excluded from receiving the vaccination were removed.
  - Medical records of all patients meeting inclusion criteria were reviewed to determine if vaccinations for influenza and pneumococcal pneumonia were appropriately ordered and administered or for the presence of docu-

mentation that appropriately justified why the vaccination was not given (e.g., patient refusal).

- Data were aggregated to determine monthly compliance.

Analyze

Compliance rates were reviewed monthly by the HPSQC.

Failures were reviewed monthly with the quality improvement team and the HPSQC leadership to determine if further changes needed to be made, such as further improvements to the communications plan or adjustments to the previously existing order set.

Results

See Fig. 2.

For in-depth discussion and review of results from this project, please see the previously published article below:

Peterson S, Taylor R, Sawyer M, et al. The power of involving house staff in quality improvement. An interdisciplinary house staff- driven vaccination initiative. Am J Med Qual, first published online ahead of print May 9, 2014. doi:10.1177/1062860614532682

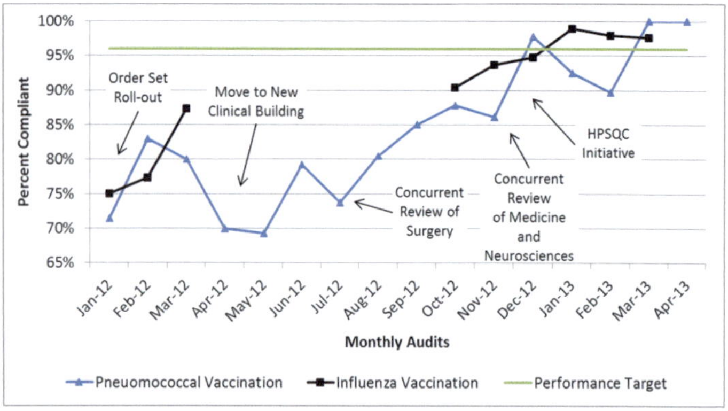

Fig. 2 Percent compliance based on monthly audits

Improve

Based on reviewed failures with the quality improvement vaccination team, subsequent changes were made to the communication plan including escalation of communication from resident to senior resident to fellow to attending for vaccinations that were ordered incorrectly.

Based on reviewed failures, minor changes were made to the order set as it was noted that the most commonly missed comorbidity requiring pneumococcal vaccination was asthma and smoking. The order of the comorbidities was changed in the order set to better highlight these common comorbidities.

Control

Compliance rates continue to be reviewed by the HPSQC leadership.

The HPSQC leadership attended the quality improvement team vaccination meetings for the year following implementation. They continue to be involved at times that are concerning for a potential drop in compliance such as the beginning of the academic year when new house staff enter the system and in the fall when influenza compliance rates begin to be tracked.

Challenges

Scope involved every inpatient department. There are a small number of departments such as oncology that have a greater fellowship involvement in addition to strong feelings about vaccination management in their patient population that had to be delicately handled.

While there were representative members from every department on the HPSQC, not every department member was present at every meeting, requiring regular email communications regarding project implementation and progress.

There was a dependence on members of the HPSQC to distribute information to their respective departments. If there was concern that we were not getting responses from a HPSQC member, program directors were carbon copied for critical messages such as the education slide set, to ensure that the information was communicated to the involved residency program.

Significant and regular participation by the HPSQC leadership in both the regular HPSQC meetings and in meetings with the institutional QI team were necessary.

Successes

This project aided the institution in reaching goal compliance rates of >96 % while adhering to CDC guidelines.

Attending Comments

An important contributor to the success of this project was the selection of a problem that aligned with the hospital's priorities for directing resources to produce improvement.

Additionally, the tenacity and interpersonal skills of the HPSQC chair, who directed the house staff effort on this project, was critical for its success.

If you have any questions about the information covered in this chapter or other medical safety and quality improvement-related topics, please contact us at http://www.medicalqualityandsafetyforum.com. The website will also provide a forum where you can ask specific questions about your safety and medical quality improvement projects or mentor upcoming medical quality leaders.

References

1. Peterson S, Taylor R, Sawyer M, et al., The power of involving house staff in quality improvement. An interdisciplinary house staff-driven vaccination initiative. Am J Med Qual, first published online ahead of print May 9, 2014. doi:10.1177/1062860614532682.
2. Kroger AT, Sumaya CV, Pickering LK, Atkinson WL. General recommendations on immunization: recommendations of the Advisory Committee on Immunization Practices (ACIP). MMWR. 2011;60(No. RR-2). Available at http://www.cdc.gov/vaccines/pubs/acip-list.htm.
3. Joint Commission on Accreditation of Health Care Organizations. Specifications manual for national hospital inpatient quality measures v4.2b. http://www.jointcommission.org/assets/1/6/HIQR_SpecsManual_v4_2bPDF4.zip. Accessed 18 Sept 2014.

Implementing Early Rehabilitation in the ICU to Improve Patient Outcomes

DMAIC Phase: *Control*

Ibtehal Kimawi and Dale M. Needham

Tools
Translating evidence into practice (TRIP), literature review

What

- Evidence: Bed rest and immobility are associated with negative outcomes, especially for critically ill patients [1, 2].
- Reality: Bed rest and immobility are widespread among critically ill patients [3–5].
- Quality gap: We need to increase patient mobility to improve patient outcomes.

The original version of this chapter was revised. An erratum to this chapter can be found at DOI 10.1007/978-3-319-24190-6_35

I. Kimawi (✉) • D. M. Needham
Department of Pulmonary and Critical Care Medicine, Johns Hopkins University School of Medicine, 1830 East Monument Street, 5th floor, Baltimore, MD 21287, USA
e-mail: ikimawi1@jhmi.edu; dale.needham@jhmi.edu

L. Atanelov (ed.), *Resident's Handbook of Medical Quality and Safety*, DOI 10.1007/978-3-319-24190-6_14

How

- We employed the translating evidence into practice (TRIP) model to structure our quality improvement (QI) project [6].
- We conducted a literature review on bed rest and its complications, as well as on the intensive care unit (ICU) mobility and its benefits, and published it [2, 7–11].
- We identified specific barriers to early mobility to tackle over approximately 1 year [12–14].
- We created a close working relationship with other stakeholders, including the directors of the medical intensive care unit (MICU), the division of pulmonary and critical care medicine, and the Department of Physical Medicine and Rehabilitation, and champions from MICU nursing, physical, and occupational therapy, respiratory therapy, and physiatry.
- We were able to ensure clinician buy-in part due, in part, to leadership of two well-respected MICU physicians leading or supporting the project and actively engaging stakeholders to understand the rationale for the QI project [14, 15].
- After review of the US federal government's Office of Human Right Protection (OHRP) guidance for quality improvement projects with an experienced chair of an institutional review board (IRB) at our institution, the project was deemed "quality improvement" and did not require formal review by the IRB or informed consent [16].
- Our intervention included reducing sedation and attempting rehabilitation, in all eligible patients, by physical and occupational therapist. We published a "how to" article specifically to help others implement their own local ICU rehabilitation QI projects [14]. The time required from planning to starting the intervention was approximately 1 year.
- Major challenges and learning points of the project included convincing hospital leaders in providing funding for this clinical work (no research funding was sought),

patients' physiological instability while critically ill, concerns about safety during rehabilitation sessions, and inadequate staffing, training, and knowledge prior to starting the project [14].

- Major successes of the project were sustained improvements, over more than 5 years, in delivering early rehabilitation and improving functional mobility of patients in our MICU [17] and beyond. Moreover, we created highly successful new conferences specifically focused on ICU rehabilitation education and research.
- Our project generated substantial media attention which contributed to both clinician and patient/family interest and knowledge in this area [18].
- We had the opportunity to further publicize our project at national and international scientific meetings, including those offered by the American Thoracic Society and the American Academy of Physical Medicine and Rehabilitation.
- Furthermore, we created an international interactive virtual community supporting ICU mobility, called the ICU Recovery Network (IRN), with more than 600 members from around the world. We also created and maintained additional educational websites: www.hopkinsmedicine.org/OACIS and www.mobilization-network.org.
- Offshoot projects were created, including evaluating the safety of physical therapy over the first 2.5 years of our critical care physical medicine and rehabilitation program, evaluating the safety of physical therapy in ICU patients with femoral catheters, and decreasing the use of sedative infusions and improving sleep quality to increase days awake without delirium [13, 19–22].
- Reflecting back, we now believe that our projects were successful due to the use of a structured QI model [6], allowing adequate time for project planning and culture change and having engaged multidisciplinary champions.

If you have any questions about the information covered in this chapter or other medical safety and quality improvement-related topics, please contact us at http://www.medicalqualityandsafetyforum.com. The website will also provide a forum where you can ask specific questions about your safety and medical quality improvement projects or mentor upcoming medical quality leaders.

References

1. Clavet H, Hebert PC, Fergusson D, Doucette S, Trudel G. Joint contracture following prolonged stay in the intensive care unit. CMAJ. 2008;178:691–7.
2. Truong AD, Fan E, Brower RG, Needham DM. Bench-to-bedside review: mobilizing patients in the intensive care unit – from pathophysiology to clinical trials. Crit Care. 2009;13:216.
3. Berney SC, Harrold M, Webb SA, et al. Intensive care unit mobility practices in Australia and New Zealand: a point prevalence study. Crit Care Resusc. 2013;15:260–5.
4. Nydahl P, Ruhl AP, Bartoszek G, et al. Early mobilization of mechanically ventilated patients: a 1-day point-prevalence study in Germany. Crit Care Med. 2014;42:1178–86.
5. Winkelman C, Higgins PA, Chen YJ. Activity in the chronically critically ill. Dimens Crit Care Nurs. 2005;24:281–90.
6. Pronovost PJ, Berenholtz SM, Needham DM. Translating evidence into practice: a model for large scale knowledge translation. BMJ. 2008;337:a1714.
7. Parker A, Sricharoenchai T, Needham DM. Early Rehabilitation in the Intensive Care Unit: Preventing Physical and Mental Health Impairments. Curr Phys Med Rehabil Rep. 2013;1:307–14.
8. Stevens RD, Dowdy DW, Michaels RK, Mendez-Tellez PA, Pronovost PJ, Needham DM. Neuromuscular dysfunction acquired in critical illness: a systematic review. Intensive Care Med. 2007;33:1876–91.
9. Desai SV, Law TJ, Needham DM. Long-term complications of critical care. Crit Care Med. 2011;39:371–9.
10. Needham DM. Mobilizing patients in the intensive care unit: improving neuromuscular weakness and physical function. JAMA. 2008;300:1685–90.

11. Korupolu R, Gifford J, Needham DM. Early mobilization of critically ill patients: reducing neuromuscular complications after intensive care. Contem Crit Care. 2009;6:1–12.
12. Zanni JM, Korupolu R, Fan E, et al. Rehabilitation therapy and outcomes in acute respiratory failure: an observational pilot project. J Crit Care. 2010;25:254–62.
13. Hager DN, Dinglas VD, Subhas S, et al. Reducing deep sedation and delirium in acute lung injury patients: a quality improvement project. Crit Care Med. 2013;41:1435–42.
14. Needham DM, Korupolu R. Rehabilitation quality improvement in an intensive care unit setting: implementation of a quality improvement model. Top Stroke Rehabil. 2010;17:271–81.
15. Hopkins RO, Spuhler VJ, Thomsen GE. Transforming ICU culture to facilitate early mobility. Crit Care Clin. 2007;23:81–96.
16. Needham DM, Korupolu R, Zanni JM, et al. Early physical medicine and rehabilitation for patients with acute respiratory failure: a quality improvement project. Arch Phys Med Rehabil. 2010;91:536–42.
17. Dinglas VD, Parker AM, Reddy DR, et al. A quality improvement project sustainably decreased time to onset of active physical therapy intervention in acute lung injury patients. Ann Am Thorac Soc. 2014;11(8):1230–8.
18. Gina Kolata. New idea to cut ICU trauma: get patients up, tubes and all. The New York Times, January 11, 2009. A2.
19. Damluji A, Zanni JM, Mantheiy E, Colantuoni E, Kho ME, Needham DM. Safety and feasibility of femoral catheters during physical rehabilitation in the intensive care unit. J Crit Care. 2013;28(4):535.
20. Kamdar BB, Yang J, King LM et al. Developing, implementing, and evaluating a multifaceted quality improvement intervention to promote sleep in an ICU. Am J Med Qual. 2013;29(6): 546–554.
21. Sricharoenchai T, Parker AM, Zanni JM, Nelliot A, Dinglas VD, Needham DM. Safety of physical therapy interventions in critically ill patients: a single-center prospective evaluation of 1110 intensive care unit admissions. J Crit Care. 2014;29:395–400.
22. Kamdar BB, King LM, Collop NA, et al. The effect of a quality improvement intervention on perceived sleep quality and cognition in a medical ICU. Crit Care Med. 2013;41:800–9.

Developing a Consistent Multidisciplinary Delivery of Therapy Care System for Acute Care Therapy Services

DMAIC Phase: Improve

Julie Kreif

> **Tools**
> DMAIC (Define, Measure, Analyze, Improve, and Control) five-step approach to improvement
> SBAR (Situation, Background Assessment, Recommendation) communication tool

J. Kreif, PT, MBA (✉)
Department of Physical Medicine and Rehabilitation, The John Hopkins Hospital, 1800 Orleans Street, Meyer 2-109, Baltimore 21287, MD, USA
e-mail: jkreif1@jhmi.edu

L. Atanelov (ed.), *Resident's Handbook of Medical Quality and Safety*, DOI 10.1007/978-3-319-24190-6_15

Project Motivation (**SBAR***)

Situation

What

- Acute care therapy services employ a large number of new graduate physical therapists (PTs), occupational therapists (OTs), and speech-language pathologists (SLPs).
- PTs, OTs, and SLPs are responsible for determining the frequency of therapy visits for adult acute care inpatients.
- But, therapists are inconsistent in determining the frequency of acute care therapy visits which results in variation with treatment frequency with comparable inpatient conditions.

How

- Observation from clinical experience, treatment review, and documentation review
- Feedback from inpatient customers, therapy staff, and hospital health-care team members

Background

What

- Inconsistencies among therapy staff in determining the frequency of inpatient therapy visits
- Health-care provider, caregiver, and inpatient complaints related to frequency of therapy visits
- Variation among hospital units regarding the role of acute care therapy (PTs, OTs, SLPs) versus other health-care providers versus family with inpatient care

How

- Observation from clinical experience, treatment review, and documentation review
- Feedback from inpatient customers, therapy staff, and hospital health-care team members
- Patient and caregiver grievances reported to Patient Relations Department

Assessment

- Acute care therapy practice of determining the frequency of inpatient visits is inconsistent and lacks a framework for decision-making.
- Therapy staff will require ongoing education and training to improve practice.
- Non-therapy hospital health-care providers and caregivers will be beneficial to augment therapy plan of care and thus supplement inpatient activity and mobility.

Recommendations

- Develop a framework for delivery of therapy care that helps delineate frequency, educate customers on the framework, and train therapy staff on the framework, *in order to*
- Increase consistency in therapy delivery of care, to decrease variation in therapy visit frequency and involve non-therapy care providers and caregivers in the therapy plan of care, *utilizing*
- Existing therapy multidisciplinary staffing structure consisting of acute care leadership (manager, two team leaders), service leadership (six team coordinators), and staff development roles (three clinical specialists) to provide input into framework development and help train therapy and tech staff of 85, *and utilizing*
- Existing acute care therapy competency training system for onboarding new staff and maintaining competence of existing staff members

Project Implementation (**DMAIC***)

Define

- Problem: No framework to guide therapy staff in determining frequency of acute care therapy visits.
- Goal: Create an algorithm for therapy care delivery and training materials for all therapy disciplines (PTs, OTs, SLPs) as well as non-therapy health-care providers.

- Benefit: Improved communication and expectations regarding delivery of therapy care and frequency of therapy visits in the acute care setting.
- Scope: All adult acute care therapy staff and adult inpatient units.

Measure

What

- Frequency of acute care therapy visits
- Create an algorithm to document visit frequency levels and measure compliance with the documentation.

How

- Train acute care therapy staff with small group classes, online modules, direct observation, and document review to determine appropriate patient level at the time of therapy evaluation.
- Audit therapy staff compliance with algorithm visit frequency levels by documentation audit and observation.
- Create an algorithm with visit frequency levels based primarily upon the difference between a patient's current functional status and their functional baseline.
- Develop an algorithm with therapist input that addresses the acute care patient populations treated by therapy.
    - A multidisciplinary therapy group determined functional levels to correspond with frequency of visits and an algorithm to support practice.
    - The algorithm was tailored to the following patient populations for which therapy is consulted:
        - PT general
        - PT cardiopulmonary (non-CF)
        - PT specialty
        - OT general
        - OT specialty
        - SLP dysphagia management

    - SLP cognition/language/motor speech and communication disorders
    - SLP tracheostomy management

- Develop an algorithm that simplifies decision-making when determining the visit frequency for follow-up therapy care.
  - The algorithm identified the following frequency levels based upon the patient's functional variance from baseline (see example):

Example: PT general algorithm for delivery of therapy care (Table 1)

- Train therapy staff (79) and rehab techs (6) for implementation. Acute care leadership (manager, team leader) taught a small group class, including lecture and case study, for consistency of message. Service leadership, team coordinators (TC), and clinical specialists (CS) provided direct observation experiences for modeling. Staff completed independent study with online modules and quiz. Acute care leadership ultimately reviewed materials and staff performance for competency completion with each staff member.
- Create a delivery of care competency for therapy staff completion and for ongoing training as new staff are hired (see example).

See Fig. 1: initial delivery of care for acute care therapy competency, for example.

- Engage nursing staff and care providers with therapy delivery of care algorithm and importance of hospital health-care providers and caregiver involvement in carrying out the therapy plan of care.
  - Therapy leadership met individually with each nurse manager to share materials which included definitions, goals, explanation of therapy levels, etc. Some service lines identified additional groups for education, such as physician assistants.

Table 1 Example of algorithm for delivery of general physical therapy care

PT	General algorithm		
Evaluation	Therapy plan of care for patient	Functional status of patient	Ongoing intervention
Level 0	Provided with any of the following resources for patient, family, and unit staff to implement: care team instructions, activity/mobility plan, educational handouts, exercises, and/or worksheets Provided with activity calendar to track and reinforce the importance of daily activity performed by the patient Provided with activity status form to inform caregivers and/or unit staff of abilities Receive a discharge recommendation	Patient at functional baseline and does not have skilled therapy needs. Patient presents with 0 % or 100 % of disability per AMPAC [1] 6-clicks score	Discharged from therapy care
Level 1	As above and in addition: Follow-up sessions may be in the acute care clinic (if deemed appropriate for transport)	Patient near functional baseline or requires contact guard or supervision	Visit 1–2 times per week until patient progresses to independent activity at preadmission/pre-op level
Level 2	As above and in addition: Follow-up sessions may be bedside or in acute care clinic, depending on patient goals	Patient not at functional baseline and requires minimum to moderate assistance	Visit 3–4 times per week until patient progresses to Level 1
Level 3	As above and in addition: Follow-up sessions may be bedside or in acute care clinic, depending on patient goals and amount of assistance required	Patient not at functional baseline and requires maximum assistance	Visit 5–7 times per week until patient progresses to Level 2

JOHNS HOPKINS MEDICINE

Department of Physical Medicine and Rehabilitation

Physical Therapy / Occupational Therapy / Speech Language Pathology
Osler 1-159/ Meyer 2-109
600 North Wolfe Street
Baltimore, MD 21287-8319
410-955-6214/ 410-955-6758

Staff Member:____

Acute Care Services Delivery of Care Learning Packet Check-Off

Expectation	Completed (Date)	Comments
1. Review service specific presentation and algorithms for provision of therapy care specific to service. (TL/Mgr)		
2. Review algorithm for provision of co-treatment. (TL/Mgr)		
3. Review "Discharge Planning for ACS" (CS/TC)		
4. Documentation (3 samples) reflects correct leveling for patients.		
5. Shadow (3x) rounds coverage with TC or CS.		
6. Observation of staff member at rounds reflects proactive communication for therapy.		
7. Complete mylearning module "Teach Back Patient Education Method v. 1.0"		
8. Complete mylearning module "Multidisciplinary Rounds"		
9. Complete mylearning module "JHH Care Coordination"		
10. Complete learning packet quiz.		

Staff Member Signature:____________________________________

TC/CS/TL Signature:______________________________________
4/2014

Fig. 1 Initial delivery of care for acute care therapy competency

- Therapy staff completed tools (in patient room) which identified patient's activity status (in nursing-friendly terminology), goals, and activity progress (see example).
- Therapy staff reinforced the inpatient's functional status at daily care coordination rounds (Fig. 2).

JOHNS HOPKINS MEDICINE

Activity Status

Patient Name: ______________ Date: ____________ Level: __________

Precautions/Weight Bearing: ______________________________

Bed Mobility: ______________________________

Transfers: Sit to stand: ____________ Into chair: ______________

Equipment needed: ______________________________

Walking: ______________________________

Equipment needed: ______________________________

Inside Room ☐ With staff ☐

Hallways ☐ With family members ☐

KEY

Person assist: *1 or 2 person*
Lift: *Use of Arjo lift for transfer*
Lateral transfer: *Use of pull across method into cardiac or bariatric chair*

Maximal Assist: *Performs less than 25% of task*
Moderate Assist: *Performs about 50% of task*
Minimal Assist: *Performs more than 75% of task*
Contact Guard: *Requires hands-on assist for guidance*
Supervision: *No hands-on assist required but should not perform the task alone*
Set-up: *Requires set-up for task but can perform task alone*
Independent: *Performs task alone*

Activities of Daily Living: Toileting: Bedside Commode ☐ Toilet ☐

	Assistance	Position	Equipment
Grooming			
Upper Body Bathing			
Upper Body Dressing			
Lower Body Bathing			
Lower Body Dressing			
Feeding			

DO NOT THROW AWAY - WIPE CLEAN WITH CAVI WIPES!

FIG. 2 Patient activity status form

Analyze

What

- Analyze therapy compliance with algorithm visit frequency levels.

How

- Regular meetings of service leadership with acute care leadership to discuss inconsistencies with algorithm visit frequency levels between six acute care therapy services: cardiac, medicine, ICU, neurosciences, surgery, and medical/surgical oncology. Variation with visit frequencies was quickly identified and could be examined on a case-by-case basis to determine follow-up, such as education with individual therapists or a service line.
- Regular meetings of therapy team coordinators with nurse managers to discuss challenges and identify barriers with implementing therapy plan of care.

Improve

- Identified need for re-training acute care therapy staff and created a follow-up delivery of care competency checkoff for completion by acute care leadership after therapy staff have been practicing for 6 months (see example).

See Fig. 3: follow-up delivery of care for acute care therapy competency, for example.

Control

Stage not reached yet

Challenges

- Lack of an existing cross-disciplinary algorithm to guide therapy practice in the area of visit frequency
- Changing the expectation of health-care providers in the acute care setting that therapy provides all-patient activity and mobility
- Ongoing consistency with a large acute care therapy staff in determining the frequency level for inpatients
- Consistent messaging with patient- and family-centered care to increase those individuals' involvement with appropriate patient care

JOHNS HOPKINS MEDICINE

Department of Physical Medicine and Rehabilitation

Physical Therapy / Occupational Therapy / Speech Language Pathology
Osler 1-159/ Meyer 2-109
600 North Wolfe Street
Baltimore, MD 21287-8319
410-955-6214/ 410-955-6758

Staff Member:____

Acute Care Services Delivery of Care Competency Check-Off

Expectation	Completed (Date)	Comments
1. Review materials on AMPAC 6 clicks specific to service. (TC/TL/Supv)		
2. Observation of staff member at rounds and following behaviors are noted:		
- Facilitation of mobility or activity data reporting with majority of patients		
- Proactive questioning re. patients functional status as a form of screening		
- Appropriate redirection of unnecessary therapy services		
- Staff education re. resources, tips when necessary		
- Appropriate discharge recommendations		
- Proactive care coordination to improve acute care treatment		
- Effectively uses strategies to optimize efficiency (ex. POE, updated comments, etc)		
3. Documentation (2 samples) reflects correct leveling for patients and provider instructions.		

Staff Member Signature:____

TC/CS/TL/Supv Signature:____
4/2014

FIG. 3 Follow-up delivery of care for acute care therapy competency

Successes

- Created better alignment of acute care therapy services with those inpatients that have greater functional needs and would benefit from skilled therapy

- Partnered with another department initiative, activity and mobility promotion, to facilitate a culture change with hospital units to increase inpatient mobility and activity
- Improved patient, caregiver, and hospital health-care provider awareness of the patient's abilities and readiness for discharge due to increased involvement of the care team during the patient's hospital stay
- Discovered how influential a team of therapists and rehab techs can be when they are engaged and presenting a uniform message to customers (health-care team members, patients, and caregivers)

If you have any questions about the information covered in this chapter or other medical safety and quality improvement-related topics, please contact us at http://www.medicalqualityandsafetyforum.com. The website will also provide a forum where you can ask specific questions about your safety and medical quality improvement projects or mentor upcoming medical quality leaders.

References

1. Jette A, Haley SM, Coster W, Ni Peng. Boston University Activity Measure for Post-Acute Care (AM-PAC). Instruction manual. 5/20/2014.

Quality Improvement and CAUTI Project: A Nursing Approach

PDCA Phase: *Act*

Amber Renaud

> **Tools**
> PDCA

Nurses provide direct patient care and are key members in contributing to quality improvement. A multidisciplinary approach is essential to the application of performance improvement in a hospital setting. There are multiple levels of QI councils for nurses, starting at the unit level and then continuing upward through the hierarchy to hospital and corporate levels. These councils, manned mostly by nurses, follow a PDCA – Plan, Do, Check, Act – approach when performing data collection to initiate changes in practice. This data is collected from, among other places, patients' medical records, quality control, and staff and research studies. It is a continuous process that is peer-reviewed. Data is collected only by certified and trained nurses and then submitted to the

A. Renaud (✉)
Department of Rehabilitation, MedStar Good Samaritan Hospital, 9009 Fieldchat Road, Nottingham, MD 21236, USA
e-mail: a.sentzrn@hotmail.com

L. Atanelov (ed.), *Resident's Handbook of Medical Quality and Safety*, DOI 10.1007/978-3-319-24190-6_16

council leaders. To maintain confidentiality, the use of medical record numbers is in place of patient identifiers.

The main projects that nursing quality and safety councils work on include Catheter Associated Urinary Tract Infection (CAUTI), Healthcare Acquired Pressure Ulcers (HAPU), pain assessment, infection prevention, and fall prevention. As a result to using the PDCA approach in combination with our applied research, changes to nursing policies and practices have come about that have improved the overall quality of care of our patients. HAPU and CAUTI rates have drastically declined, and more members of the health- care team are contributing to fall prevention and pain management than in previous years.

It is my strong belief that a nurse's approach to contributing to the overall QI of a hospital facility is quintessential. Nurses can provide critical direct research, such as CAUTI, while also implementing better quality through unique practices. This is all highlighted by using a PDCA nursing approach.

Plan

The first step of the PDCA approach was initiated by a plan to collect a variety of data on urinary catheters. This was done to assess the amount of CAUTI that has the potential to be preventable and to initiate a change in practice in order to drastically reduce, or eliminate, CAUTI infections all together. The data collected includes information on Foley insertion dates, bag placement, amount of urine in the bag at a random check, and other measurable actualities. The data was to be collected on a monthly basis from the members of the Quality and Safety Hospital Council. Information from the data collection then needed to be written on a formatted standardized handout to which each nurse physically assessed the patient's urinary catheter and performed an electronic as well as a tangible chart review.

Do

The next step in the process started with the nursing process of information assessment, implementation, and evaluation. A collaboration with other nurses occurred secondary to similar interest in order to reach the goal. We performed interventions on a small scale that included removing Foley catheters on day one or two post insertion and educated staff on the project. Another intervention involved having the catheter distributor come into the hospital and review proper placement and protocol that specifically related to the brand that our hospital uses. With the help of the professional practice council, who devised a nurse-driven protocol, a change was made to our practice. A new policy came about that states nurses no longer need a physician's order to discontinue an indwelling urinary catheter. Exceptions include those catheters placed via urologist.

Check

The third step was to analyze our preliminary data. We found that with an increase in auditing, open communication to physicians, and awareness to staff of the project, there was a decline in the amount of CAUTIs. The preliminary final results starting with the first quarter went from 1.2 to 0 in the second quarter (number of infections/urinary catheter days × 1000).

Act

The final step in the process is to continue to implement evidenced-based practices to prevent indwelling catheter-associated urinary tract infections. We applied the interventions as previously stated and will continue semiannual Foley catheter audits and monthly CAUTI audits to evaluate the effectiveness of the continued interventions.

Challenges to this project included limited amount of time to complete the audits and standardizing the audit tool. Other barriers included getting all members of the healthcare team onboard and aware of the project and arranging a time for staff to be reeducated on the correct practice of Foley placement.

Successes encountered during this project contain a variety of sources. The first and most obvious is the actual reduction in the CAUTI rate and that supports our goal accomplishment. Other success includes the empowerment of nurses to be more autonomous which in turn increases morale on the unit. The teamwork involved providing an open communication in the workplace, and it is because of all the team members contribution that the project was a success.

In addition to research, as stated, nurses have unique practices that can implement quality improvement because they make up the front line of patient care. It is imperative that all members of the health-care team remember that QI is a multidisciplinary action that the patient, and their families, can benefit from by all of us working collectively.

If you have any questions about the information covered in this chapter or other medical safety and quality improvement-related topics, please contact us at http://www.medicalqualityandsafetyforum.com. The website will also provide a forum where you can ask specific questions about your safety and medical quality improvement projects or mentor upcoming medical quality leaders.

Streamlining the Stat Medication Process: An Interdisciplinary Quality Improvement Project

DMAIC Phase: Improve

Melinda D. Sawyer, Jennifer V. Gillespie, Denice L. Duda, and Robert E. Hody

M.D. Sawyer (✉)
Armstrong Institute for Patient Safety and Quality, John Hopkins University School of Medicine, 600 Wolfe Street, Carnegie 667, Baltimore, MD 21287, USA
e-mail: msawyer1@jhmi.edu

J.V. Gillespie
Department of Pharmacy, The Johns Hopkins Hospital, 600 North Wolfe Street/Carnegie 180, Baltimore, MD 21287-6180, USA
e-mail: jkacmar1@jhmi.edu

D.L. Duda
Department of Quality Improvement, The John Hopkins Hospital, 600 N. Wolfe St, Baltimore, MD 21287, USA
e-mail: darthur2@jhmi.edu

R.E. Hody
Armstrong Institute for Patient Safety and Quality, John Hopkins University School of Medicine, 750 East Pratt Street, 15th Floor, Baltimore, MD 21202, USA
e-mail: rhody@jhmi.edu

L. Atanelov (ed.), *Resident's Handbook of Medical Quality and Safety*, DOI 10.1007/978-3-319-24190-6_17

Tools
SBAR: Previously described in other cases, DMAIC: Previously described in other cases, Value Stream Mapping, Root causes, modifiable and non-modifiable, variations in time

Value Stream Mapping

A value stream helps you see and understand the flow of a product through a process. This includes the actions that are value added and non-value added [1]. Using value stream mapping means evaluating and improving the entire process and not just improving the individual steps within a process [1].

- Use a paper and pencil to draw each step within a value stream.
- Start with the customer (e.g., patient) and work backward to the start of the production process.
- In the example below, we performed direct observations to understand time through each process and to identify wasted time within the process.
- Evaluate the current state of the value stream map for opportunities to reduce non-value-added processes or improve value-added processes.
- Draw a "future state" value stream map of an ideal process.
- In the example below, we again performed direct observations to analyze how our interventions (changes to the value stream map) impacted the value stream.

Project Motivation (**SBAR***)

Situation

What

- Stat medications, from the Latin *statim*, meaning immediately, are reserved for the highest priority orders and life-threatening situations that must be administered within a limited time frame [2, 3].
- Hospital policy states stat medications are to be administered within 30 min from the time the medication is ordered by a provider.

How

- A survey of the Department of Medicine general medical unit and medical progressive care unit nurses ($n = 156$) revealed their number one challenge in the medication use process was medications arriving late or never arriving from the pharmacy.
- Medications ordered stat were of most concern due to the urgency related to the patients' deteriorating condition.

Background

What

- A previous phase (DMAIC phase: measure) of this project included **value stream mapping***, which included measuring time within each phase of the medication use process. These measures were obtained through observations of medications through this process. Results ($n = 33$) included (in minutes):
  - Time from stat order entered to pharmacist verification: mean 17, max 117
  - Time from pharmacist verification to pharmacy technician preparation: mean 8, max 46
  - Time from pharmacy technician preparation to medication checked by pharmacist: mean 1, max 5

  - Time from medication checked by pharmacist to medication delivered to the unit: mean 14, max 84
  - Time from medication delivered to the unit to the RN locating the medication: mean 15, max 52
  - Time from the RN locating the medication to the RN administering the medication to the patient: mean 15, max 74
  - Total: Only one out of 33 stat medication observations met the 30-min turnaround time (3 %).

- Variations in time through each step of the medication use process have multiple root causes.
- Several of these root causes are modifiable while others are not. Examples of each type are:

  - Modifiable – lack of a notification system to indicate to health-care worker (pharmacist, pharmacy technician, nurse) that a stat medication is in the queue
  - Non-modifiable – patient characteristics such as loss of intravenous access at the same time as medication arrival on unit

How

- Observations of 33 stat medications in prior phase of project

Assessment

- Stat medications are reserved for life-threatening situations and must be administered within a limited time frame.
- Significant delays in administering stat medications are not acceptable and can be dangerous.

Recommendations

- Reduce the turnaround time (time from medication order to administration of medication to patient) for stat medications.
- Reduce the number of steps in the stat medication use process without compromising patient safety.

Project Implementation (**DMAIC***)

Define

- Problem: Significant delays in stat medication administration can be dangerous to patients.
- Goal: Increase the number of stat medications that meet the 30-min turnaround time from 3 % to 50 %.
- Benefit: Reduce unintended consequences that result from delays in medication administration during life-threatening situations.
- Scope: 11 inpatient units (eight inpatient medical units, one medical progressive care unit, two general neurology/neurosurgical units).

Measure

- Measure time through each phase of the medication use process (described above) for stat medications both before and after implementation of an intervention.
- Measure the percent of stat medications that are administered within 30 min of the time it is ordered before and after implementation of an intervention.

Analyze

What

- Analyze differences in time through each phase of the medication use process.
- Analyze differences in the proportion of stat medications that are administered within 30 min of the time it is ordered.

How

- One-way ANOVA was used to compare changes in time through each phase of the medication use process.
- Fisher's exact test was used to compare the difference in proportions of stat medications that were administered within 30 min of the time it was ordered.

Improve

What

- Pharmacists and nurses reviewed the modifiable and non-modifiable root causes of delays and selected to reduce the number of steps of the medication use process for the most frequently ordered stat medications.
- This was achievable without compromising any safety checks or procedures.
- Steps in the stat medication use process prior to intervention: current state value stream map (Fig. 1)
- Steps in the stat medication process after the intervention: future state value stream map (Fig. 2)

How

- In each unit, automated dispensing cabinets (Pyxis® MedStation) are in the medication room to store and lock narcotics and various other medications.

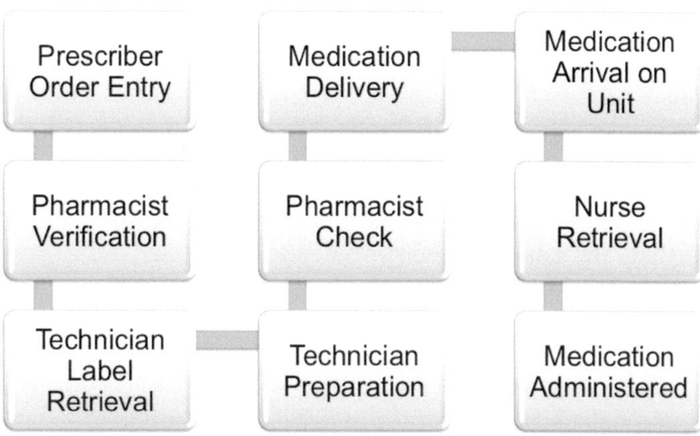

Fig. 1 Steps in the stat medication use process prior to intervention (current state value stream map)

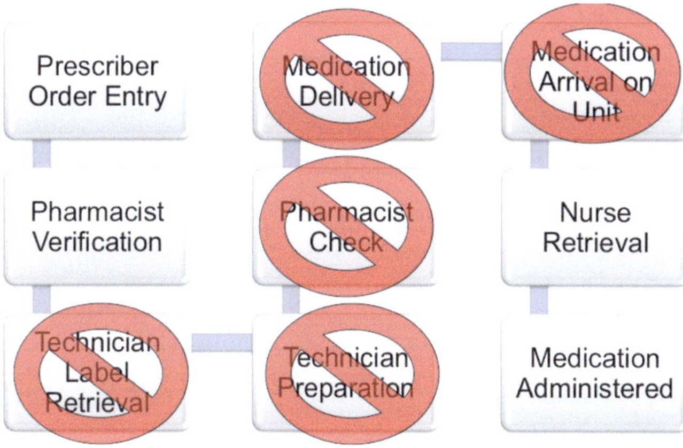

FIG. 2 Steps in the stat medication use process after the intervention (future state value stream map)

- These automated dispensing cabinets (ADCs) require a pharmacist's review of the medication after which the pharmacist adds the medication to the individual patient's profile within the ADC computer.
- Within the ADC, the nurse can access medications by selecting the patient's name and selecting which medication she wishes to administer.
- Based on the availability of space with each ADC, the team identified that 41 additional medications could be added.

- All stat medication orders ($n=23{,}032$) over a 3-month period were reviewed for each individual unit to identify the 41 most frequently ordered stat medications.
  - Trends were identified for medications within each unit, within each department, and across the two departments to identify stat medications to be added to the ADC.
  - A stat medication list was developed for each unit and those medications were added to the ADC.

- This list of stat medications was taken to the Pharmacy Practice Management committee for approval to be added to the ADC. This is required by hospital policy.
- Appropriate stock levels were determined based on the frequency of stat medication order to minimize out-of-stock occurrences.
- Education was provided to all appropriate pharmacists, nurses, and physicians regarding this practice change.
  - Education included a list of the medications that would now be available in the unit ADC.

Results

Overall results:

(Figures 3 and 4)

Changes in time through steps of the medication use process:

(Figures 5 and 6)

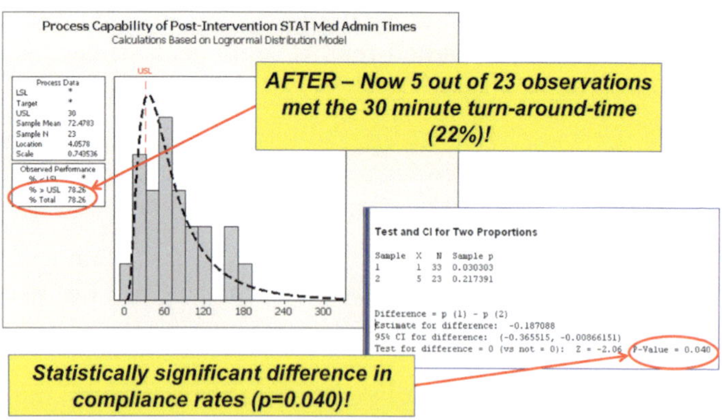

FIG. 3 Impact of intervention on 30-min turnaround time

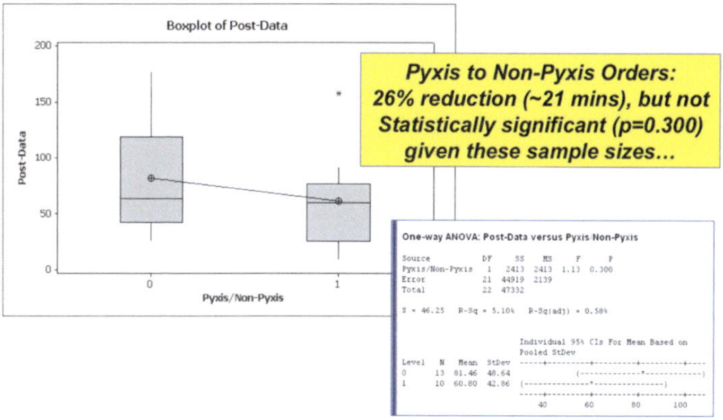

FIG. 4 Post-intervention comparison of turnaround time for medications added to the ADC (Pyxis) compared to medications not added to the ADC (non-Pyxis)

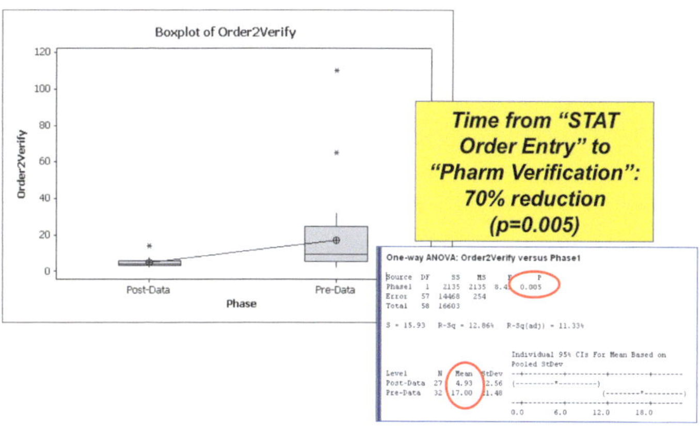

FIG. 5 Change in turnaround time for the subprocess "time from stat order entry to pharmacy verification" from pre- to post-intervention

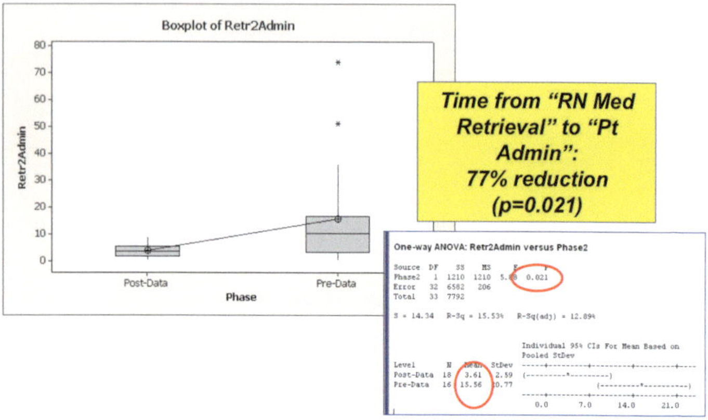

FIG. 6 Change in turnaround time for the subprocess "time from RN retrieval of medication to patient-administered medication" from pre- to post-intervention

Control

What

- ADCs have been increased from one tower to four towers, which significantly increased the number of medications that are available in the ADC on the unit.
- ADCs now have 80–95 % of all ordered medications, not just stat medications, available through this process.

Challenges

- This intervention did not change the process for all stat medications.
  - Since only 41 medications were added to the ADC, many stat medications were still prepared in the pharmacy.
  - Despite having a list posted in the medication room, nurses often reported being confused as to where to find the stat medication.

- Many root causes for delays were not addressed in this intervention due to lack of feasibility.

Successes

- Multidisciplinary collaboration between pharmacists and nurses greatly impacted the adoption of this intervention by both groups.
  - Throughout the project, frontline nurses and pharmacists from all areas were included in key decisions.

If you have any questions about the information covered in this chapter or other medical safety and quality improvement-related topics, please contact us at http://www.medicalqualityandsafetyforum.com. The website will also provide a forum where you can ask specific questions about your safety and medical quality improvement projects or mentor upcoming medical quality leaders.

References

1. Rother M, Shook J. Learning to see: value stream mapping to add value and eliminate muda. Cambridge, MA: Taylor & Francis; 2003. p. 102.
2. Jaffe A, Levine J, Citrome L. "Stat" medication administration predicts hospital discharge. Psychiatr Q. 2009;80(2):65–73.
3. Fahimi F, Sahraee Z, Amini S. Evaluation of stat orders in a teaching hospital: a chart review. Clin Drug Investig. 2011;31(4):231–5.

Part IV
Consuming and Producing Academic Literature

Publishing Your Work: A Bird's-Eye View Outline

Levi (Levan) Atanelov

> **Tools**
> PubMed database, IMRAD format, RefWorks software

1. Figure out what you want to do.
   (a) Are you on track for an academic position?
   (b) Are you publishing to get a residency/fellowship position?
   (c) Which field of medicine interests you?
   (d) What research experience do you have?
2. Find a mentor/principal investigator.
   (a) Senior mentors may have more research funding and connections that help publish faster, but they may have larger labs and may not be available for much personal time. Their reputation may help procure a better academic position in the future.
   (b) Junior mentors will be more available, but may have little funding or experience and you may have to do lots of self-learning and troubleshooting of how to get things done without funding.

L. Atanelov (✉)
Department of Physical Medicine and Rehabilitation,
Johns Hopkins Hospital, Baltimore, MD, USA
e-mail: leviatanelov@gmail.com

L. Atanelov (ed.), *Resident's Handbook of Medical Quality and Safety*, DOI 10.1007/978-3-319-24190-6_18

(c) Find mentors.

  (i) University/academic institution websites
  (ii) PubMed with filters on field of your interest and local academic institution
  (iii) Word of mouth
  (iv) Cold call, e.g., knock on the door of the lab and ask if they are looking for someone (this is more for undergrads usually).

(d) Pick a mentor that you personally get along with, research may take long time and may be hard at times, you want to make sure you are comfortable with the person you work with.

3. Find a project.

   (a) One may want to have a project first, but I recommend finding a good mentor first and perhaps doing whatever project that they have already ongoing.

      (i) They are already interested in that project, so you don't have to sell them on yours.
      (ii) It often takes a long time to get an IRB (institutional review board) approval (sometimes 1–2 years), and they already may have one for their project and you may not want to wait for 2 years to get your IRB approved.
      (iii) They may already have funding for their project.
      (iv) They may have more expertise with their project.

4. Review the literature.

   (a) Search on PubMed for review articles.
   (b) Ask your mentor to suggest key articles relevant to the research you are doing.
   (c) Pay careful attention to the methods section, as how to do these types of projects is described there and odds are your project will be a variation of the methods described in related articles.
   (d) Systematically keep track of what you read; as a low tech option, on a piece of paper, write down the title

of the article and first author and summarize some of the key points that you find salient so you can come back to these later.

5. Learn the skills/concepts relevant to the field.
    (a) This may take a while and may include training in bench work ("wet lab"), statistics, informatics, etc. Plan for having a steep learning curve, so start early.
6. Develop a hypothesis.
    (a) Develop a hypothesis that can be measured and tested within a clear time period.
    (b) Ask your mentor to formulate the hypothesis.
    (c) There are lots of online resources, but no clear definitive guide to my knowledge, see what works best for you.
7. Do the work: assume that the work will take at least a year before your work is publishable.
8. Write it up.
    (a) Follow IMRAD format.
        (i) Introduction: introduce background to the work, what has been done so far in the field, and how your work fills in the gaps.
        (ii) Methods: based on the type of research done, include appropriate methodology.
        (iii) Results
        (iv) Discussion/Conclusion
    (b) See [1] for instruction on how to publish QI articles.
    (c) Learn to use a software like RefWorks to keep track of all the references as you edit the article.
    (d) You may need an expert statistician as part of the project, find one in advance.
9. Submit.
    (a) Identify which journal you want to submit to based on **what types of articles** they have published there before and the **quality of research they normally expect.**

(b) Journals are ranked based on impact factor, high-impact-factor journals like *Science* and *New England Journal of Medicine* are more competitive.
(c) Often they will ask you to suggest reviewers for your article, be prepared to suggest people.
(d) Please don't try to submit last minute, it may take a few days to get all the information in place and get all the authors to submit their demographic data. This is important because some abstracts submitted to national conferences have deadlines for submission. Keep that in mind.

10. Revise.

(a) Editors will always have comments, this is normal.
(b) Medical research is peer-reviewed, that means other people who are also experts in your field will review and criticize your work.
(c) They may be doing the same project and may give unfair criticism, be prepared for competitive people's comments.
(d) Be prepared to submit upon request all of the data that you generated and are not showing in the publication (e.g., statistical calculations, data not presented, etc.).
(e) You will probably need to make revisions to the article which may take several months at times, be aware of that.
(f) Be polite in your comments, editors are also people and have feelings.

11. Publish.

(a) Abstracts are easier to publish and take less effort, they usually have much less impact than full article publications. Usually conferences are apt to accept abstract submissions.
(b) Data shown in abstract **with significant amount of additional data** may be used in academic article.

(c) Not all work can be published, as there is a bias to only publish positive findings, FYI.

(d) Good luck. 

If you have any questions about the information covered in this chapter or other medical safety and quality improvement-related topics, please contact us at http://www.medicalqualityandsafetyforum.com. The website will also provide a forum where you can ask specific questions about your safety and medical quality improvement projects or mentor upcoming medical quality leaders.

References

1. Holzmueller C, Pronovost P. Research and reporting methodology Organising a manuscript reporting quality improvement or patient safety research. BMJ Qual Saf 2013;22(9):777–785.

Tips for Effective Literature Searching

Carrie Price

> **Tools**
> Boolean operators, database searching, PubMed database, keywords, controlled vocabulary, subject headings, MeSH terms, Embase database, field tags, PICO format, truncating, wild card, stop words, filters, advanced searching, EndNote, RefWorks, RIS format, citation manager

Conducting a literature search is the best way to see what has already been published on a topic as well as obtain evidence for clinical decision-making and future research endeavors.

The following steps will assist in building an effective literature search. While many of the examples given are for PubMed and Embase, the theory behind the searches will be applicable in any database.

When selecting databases, always start from your affiliated organization's library or digital resources page, which will allow you to access the full text when available and to make use of the organization's subscriptions.

Know How to Use Boolean Operators

- Boolean operators are words (AND, OR, NOT) used to combine terms in the search.

C. Price (✉)
Welch Medical Library, Johns Hopkins University, School of Medicine, 1900 East Monument Street, Baltimore, MD 21205, USA
e-mail: cprice17@jhmi.edu

L. Atanelov (ed.), *Resident's Handbook of Medical Quality and Safety*, DOI 10.1007/978-3-319-24190-6_19

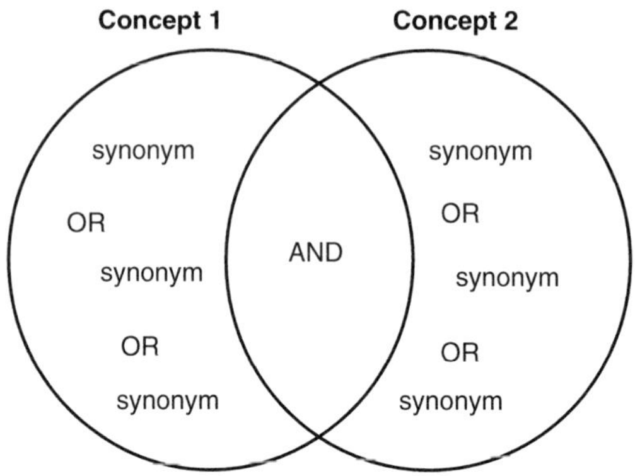

FIG. 1 Boolean operator diagram

PubMed

("physical therapy" OR "physical therapist") AND (osteoporosis) NOT child*

- Depending on how they are combined, they can increase or decrease recall (number of records).
- Use AND to combine concepts and narrow the search.
- Use OR to expand concepts and broaden the search.
- Use NOT to exclude concepts. This is used less frequently, but can still be helpful. Using NOT can exclude unwanted records:

In the example above, the searcher will find articles that discuss physical therapy AND osteoporosis, but not children.

- In the diagram below, note how OR allows the searcher to add synonyms to a concept. AND allows the searcher to locate the literature which mentions both concept one and concept two (Fig. 1). Find more on creating the search concepts in section "Now Create the Search."
- Once the searcher combines two or more concepts with AND, all future results will include only records which reference both concepts. It will exclude records which do not reference both concepts.

Keywords Versus Controlled Vocabulary

- Some databases use controlled vocabulary. These are a set list of index terms that have been applied to the record. In PubMed, the controlled vocabulary is called *Medical Subject Headings* or *MeSH*. In Embase, the controlled vocabulary is called *Emtree*.
  - For more information on MeSH: http://www.nlm.nih.gov/pubs/factsheets/mesh.html
  - For more information on Emtree: http://www.elsevier.com/online-tools/embase/about/emtree
- It is beneficial to search using both controlled vocabulary, when available, and keywords, which would include any other synonymous terms. This allows the searcher to return articles that have been indexed as well as articles that have not yet been indexed with controlled vocabulary terms.
- Keywords are synonyms associated with the concept. For example, "pediatric" is a keyword for child related. The searcher might also consider using "infant," "toddler," "baby," or "child," or "children."
- Using controlled vocabulary enables the searcher to create a very precise search. Controlled vocabulary allows the searcher to account for British versus American English, plurals, acronyms, and other ambiguities contained in the literature.
- A search using both controlled vocabulary and keywords might look something like the example below. Note the use of field tags, which are detailed in section "Use Field Tags for More Specific Results" ([MeSH] is a field tag for a MeSH term;/exp denotes an Emtree term, and [tiab] or :ti,ab commands the database to search in the title or abstract of the record):

PubMed

("Cystic Fibrosis"[Mesh] OR "cystic fibrosis"[tiab] OR "mucoviscidosis"[tiab]) AND ("Exercise Therapy"[Mesh] OR "kinesiotherapy"[tiab] OR "exercise therapy"[tiab] OR "exercise therapies"[tiab])

Embase

('cystic fibrosis'/exp or 'cystic fibrosis':ti,ab or 'mucoviscidosis':ti,ab) AND ('kinesiotherapy':ti,ab or 'kinesiotherapy':ti,ab or 'exercise therapy':ti,ab or 'exercise therapies':ti,ab)

Use Field Tags for More Specific Results

- Every database will be different, but many databases will allow the searcher to apply field tags or field descriptors to search for terms in the title, abstract, and controlled vocabulary (index terms) or to search by author, affiliation, journal, etc.
- Instructions for using each database's field tag can usually be found in the "Help" section of the database platform.
- Field tags or field descriptors assist in obtaining specific results.
- A search for a particular publication may look like this:

PubMed

(smith [au] AND hopkins [ad])
This is searching the author, Smith, with a field tag of [au] with an affiliation of Hopkins, field tag [ad].

- A search for a particular journal on a certain topic might look like this:

PubMed

jama [ta] AND "heart attack"[tiab]
The field tag [ta] is searching the journal name, while the field tag [tiab] is searching for the phrase in the title or abstract.

- A search on controlled vocabulary will look like this:

PubMed

"cystic fibrosis"[Mesh] AND "exercise therapy"[Mesh]

Embase

'cystic fibrosis'/exp AND 'kinesiotherapy'/exp
This search will only return articles that have been indexed with the controlled vocabulary terms *Cystic Fibrosis* and *Exercise Therapy* (PubMed) or *Kinesiotherapy* (Embase).

- A search for frost or frostbite and related concepts could look like this the [tiab] denotes searching in the title or abstract:

PubMed

"frost"[tiab]
But if the searcher changes the field tag, the search could return articles by the author, Frost, the [au] tag searches in the author field:

PubMed

"frost"[au]

Now Create the Search

- Write down the research question in order to get an idea of what concepts will be most relevant.
- Consider the purpose of the research. *Are you hoping to publish? Are you trying to inform a clinical decision?* This will affect how broadly you search and what type of literature you are seeking.
- Know the scope of the research. *Do you want all relevant articles on the topic, or do you want a few relevant citations?* If you want all relevant articles, you will aim to increase the recall of the search. If you want some of the most relevant citations, you will increase the precision of the search, but you may miss some pertinent articles.
- It may be helpful to use PICO to formulate the research question:

  P: Population or problem
  I: Intervention or indicator
  C: Comparison or control
  O: Outcome

- When translating your research question into PICO format, every element may not always be present. The PICO format is to assist primarily in identifying the concepts of the research question and then building on those concepts for the search. Here are a few sample questions, broken down into PICO elements:

  – How effective is baclofen pump therapy in the treatment of pediatric spasticity?

  P: pediatric spasticity
  I: baclofen pump therapy
  C: –
  O: efficacy

  – What is the best therapy program for hip fracture rehabilitation?

  P: patients with hip fractures
  I: physical therapy
  C: other kinds of therapy
  O: quality of life, range of motion, mobility, etc.

  – What's the best rehabilitation for breast-cancer-related lymphedema in breast cancer patients?

  P: breast cancer patients with lymphedema
  I: rehabilitation
  C: –
  O: quality of life, control of pain, etc.

- Once the research question is firm, begin to create search concepts.
- Think of all the terms that can describe that concept. Let's take a look at the first PICO example above:

  How effective is baclofen pump therapy in the treatment of pediatric spasticity?
  P: pediatric
  I: baclofen pump therapy
  C: –
  O: efficacy

1. First, look for a controlled vocabulary term or terms that will help narrow down to the field of pediatrics. There is both a MeSH and Emtree term for "child." There is also a MeSH and Emtree term for pediatrics. It would be helpful to include both, separated by the Boolean operator OR.
2. Next, look for a controlled vocabulary term that will identify baclofen pump therapy. There is a MeSH and Emtree term for "baclofen."
3. It is not necessary to search on "efficacy" or any outcomes. Outcomes are often not clearly stated in the title or abstract of the paper, so the searcher risks missing pertinent outcomes if limiting to specific words.
4. Make a list of synonymous terms for each concept and consider adding plurals or variations of the keywords. Place the words together with the Boolean operator OR. Enclose each concept in parentheses ().
5. Put each concept together with AND.
6. It is generally a good idea to put phrases in quotations so that the words are searched as a phrase and not as independent words.
7. Consider **truncating** a search term if it seems appropriate. For example, nurs* would catch nurse, nurses, nursing, etc.
8. Using a **wild card** can be helpful. For example, *randomi?ed* would catch *randomi<u>z</u>ed* and *randomi<u>s</u>ed*.
9. Avoid **stop words**. Stop words are words like *a*, *an*, *of*, *at*, *by*, *for*, *the*, etc. The database may have trouble reading these words and may not execute the search properly.
10. To further control the search, the searcher can choose to include or not include terms found below the term in the MeSH hierarchy. For example, Health Care Costs [MeSH] would also search on articles indexed with terms below Health Care Costs:

    Health Care Costs
        Direct Service Costs

Drug Costs
Employer Health Costs
Hospital Costs

However, the search Health Care Costs *[mesh:noexp]* commands the database to only search on that term and no other. This is called **explode** or **no explode**.

11. With controlled vocabulary terms only, our search for the example given above would look like this:

PubMed

("pediatrics"[mesh] OR "child"[mesh]) AND ("baclofen"[mesh])

Embase

('pediatrics'/exp or 'child'/exp) and ('baclofen'/exp)
This is a good search, but now consider adding keywords, which would be any synonymous terms that will identify articles that have not been indexed with controlled vocabulary terms:

PubMed

("pediatrics"[mesh] OR pediatric* OR paediatric* OR "child"[mesh] OR child*) AND ("baclofen"[mesh] OR "baclofen")

Embase

('pediatrics'/exp or pediatric* or paediatric* OR 'child'/exp OR child*) AND ('baclofen'/exp OR 'baclofen')
The second searches will have a larger number of results (higher recall) than the first searches in PubMed and Embase. The searcher could add even more terms to the first concept, such as infant, baby, neonate, adolescent, teen, etc. The term "baclofen" is unique enough to recall articles regarding baclofen treatment in the context of pump therapy.

Using Filters and Advanced Search Options

- Many searchers have a specific kind of result in mind. For example, perhaps the searcher only reads English, or is concerned with articles only published in the last 5 years, or is looking for practice guidelines.
- In PubMed, filters can be found on the left-hand side of the page after the initial search has been run.
- Other databases have similar filters in the "Advanced Search" function.
- Filtering by *date* allows the searcher to look for older or more recent material.
- Filtering by *publication type*, in many databases, allows the searcher to search for conference proceedings, clinical trials, dissertations, theses, scholarly articles, editorials, opinions, guidelines, reviews, systematic reviews, meta-analyses, and more.

More Ways to Search

- If an article seems on topic, search the reference list of the article for more articles like it. Alternatively, many databases offer citation mapping, in which you can browse articles that cite an article, or articles that were cited by the article.
- When a relevant article is found, look at its controlled vocabulary (index terms) and determine if any are worth adding to the search.
- If a journal publishes regularly on a relevant topic, consider hand searching the table of contents of recent issues to identify more material.

Save Searches

- It is advisable to create an account in databases used frequently to save searches, set up alerts and updates, and even set aside articles for future reading.
- If the searcher has created a particularly relevant search, it is a good idea to save the search for future use. Some databases allow the searcher to set up an update on a search to be emailed daily, weekly, or monthly.

Export Results

- Once the most relevant articles have been selected, databases will allow the searcher to export selected results to a bibliographic management program.
- Examples of a bibliographic management program are RefWorks and EndNote, among others.
- Many databases have a direct export function to RefWorks and EndNote.
- If using something other than RefWorks or EndNote, export to RIS format, and when importing, select "RIS format" as the option or consult the database's "Help" page for instructions on importing or exporting.

RefWorks and EndNote, Bibliographic Citation Managers

- RefWorks and EndNote allow the user to organize, store, share, and format references.
- One of the main differences between RefWorks and EndNote is that RefWorks is in the cloud (web-based) and therefore the data is available from any place the user can access the internet. EndNote is specific to the computer it has been downloaded on.

- RefWorks has a useful tool called *Write-N-Cite* that aids in creating bibliographies. This tool can be downloaded for both Windows and Mac under "Tools." For more information, see the RefWorks YouTube channel's episode on Write-N-Cite 4 (https://www.youtube.com/watch?v=um5oOxJjXAk).
- EndNote has a similar tool called *Cite While You Write*. See the EndNote user guide for more information (https://www.youtube.com/watch?v=Pa1XdyHwat4).

If you have any questions about the information covered in this chapter or other medical safety and quality improvement-related topics, please contact us at http://www.medicalqualityandsafetyforum.com. The website will also provide a forum where you can ask specific questions about your safety and medical quality improvement projects or mentor upcoming medical quality leaders.

Resources for Grading the Evidence, Appraisal, Writing, and Publishing

Carrie Price

> **Tools**
> Publication databases, evidence grading, evidence reporting, evaluating articles, publishing resources, quality improvement resources

Evidence-Based Medicine Resources

> Evidence based medicine is the conscientious, explicit, and judicious use of current best evidence in making decisions about the care of individual patients. The practice of evidence based medicine means integrating individual clinical expertise with the best available external clinical evidence from systematic research. [1]

- When searching for evidence-based literature, consider using the following databases:
  - Cumulative Index to Nursing and Allied Health Literature (CINAHL)
  - Clinical Evidence
  - Embase

C. Price (✉)
Welch Medical Library, Johns Hopkins University, School of Medicine, 1900 East Monument Street, Baltimore, MD 21205, USA
e-mail: cprice17@jhmi.edu

L. Atanelov (ed.), *Resident's Handbook of Medical Quality and Safety*, DOI 10.1007/978-3-319-24190-6_20

- PubMed's "Clinical Queries" tool (http://www.ncbi.nlm.nih.gov/pubmed/clinical)
- The Cochrane Library
- Turning Research Into Practice (TRIP)

• When grading the evidence, keep in mind the following grading schemas:

  - Grading of Recommendations Assessment, Development and Evaluation (GRADE) Working Group (http://www.gradeworkinggroup.org/)
  - US Preventive Services Task Force (http://www.uspreventiveservicestaskforce.org/uspstf/grades.htm)
  - Oxford Centre for Evidence-based Medicine Levels of Evidence(http://www.cebm.net/oxford-centre-evidence-based-medicine-levels-evidence-march-2009/)

• Additionally, consider the following standards for reporting of evidence:

  - EQUATOR Network (http://www.equator-network.org/)
  - CONSORT Statement (http://www.consort-statement.org/)
  - PRISMA Statement (http://www.prisma-statement.org/)
  - SPIRIT Statement (http://www.spirit-statement.org/)
  - SQUIRE Statement (http://squire-statement.org/)
  - TREND Statement (http://www.cdc.gov/trendstatement/)

• Critical appraisal provides a framework for evaluating individual articles to determine if the information in the article is valid and appropriate. The following tools are useful for critical appraisal:

  - Centre for Evidence-Based Medicine (http://www.cebm.net/)
  - Critical Appraisal Skills Programme (http://www.casp-uk.net)
  - Dartmouth Biomedical Libraries EBM Worksheets (http://www.dartmouth.edu/~library/biomed/guides/

research/ebm-resources-materials.html?mswitch-redir=classic)
- JAMA Series on Step-by-Step Critical Appraisal (http://www.hopkinsmedicine.org/gim/training/Osler/osler_JAMA_Steps.html)

Writing and Publishing Resources

- National Information Standards Organization (NISO) Guidelines for Structured Abstracts (http://www.niso.org/apps/group_public/download.php/6609/guidelines)
- National Library of Medicine's Journal Browser (http://www.ncbi.nlm.nih.gov/nlmcatalog/journals)
- Open Access publishers (http://oaspa.org/)
- Recommendations for the conduct, reporting, editing, and publication of scholarly work in medical journals (http://www.icmje.org/recommendations/)
- The National Library of Medicine Style Guide for Authors, Editors, and Publishers (http://www.ncbi.nlm.nih.gov/books/NBK7256/)
- US Copyright Office (http://www.copyright.gov/)
- What is a structured abstract? From National Library of Medicine (http://www.nlm.nih.gov/bsd/policy/structured_abstracts.html)

Quality Improvement Resources and Journals

When writing a quality improvement article, remember the target audience. Be sure to gather background information and expert opinion, and then detail the findings of your own project. For more information, see:

Dixon N. Writing for publication–a guide for new authors. Int J Qual Health Care. 2001;13(5):417–421. (http://intqhc.oxfordjournals.org/content/13/5/417.full.pdf)

Smith R. Quality improvement reports: a new kind of article. BMJ. 2000;321(7274):1428–1428. (http://www.ncbi.nlm.nih.gov/pmc/articles/PMC1119157/)

- The following are just a few resources are focused on quality improvement projects:
  - Agency for Healthcare Research and Quality (http://www.qualityindicators.ahrq.gov/)
  - *American Journal of Medical Quality* (http://ajm.sagepub.com/)
  - *BMJ Quality & Safety* (http://qualitysafety.bmj.com/)
  - *BMJ Quality Improvement Reports* (http://qir.bmj.com/)
  - *Health and Quality of Life Outcomes* (http://www.hqlo.com/)
  - Health Resources and Services Administration (http://www.hrsa.gov/quality/toolbox/)
  - *Joint Commission Journal on Quality and Patient Safety* (http://www.jcrinc.com/The-Joint-Commission-Journal-on-Quality-and-Patient-Safety/)
  - *Journal of Evaluation in Clinical Practice* (http://onlinelibrary.wiley.com/journal/10.1111/(ISSN)1365-2753)
  - *Journal for Healthcare Quality* (http://onlinelibrary.wiley.com/journal/10.1111/%28ISSN%291945-1474)
  - *Journal of Nursing Care Quality* (http://journals.lww.com/jncqjournal/pages/default.aspx)
  - *Journal of Public Health Management and Practice* (http://journals.lww.com/jphmp/Pages/default.aspx)
  - *Quality in Primary Care* (http://ingentaconnect.com/content/rmp/qpc)
  - *Quality Management in Healthcare* (http://journals.lww.com/qmhcjournal/pages/default.aspx)

If you have any questions about the information covered in this chapter or other medical safety and quality improvement-related topics, please contact us at http://www.medicalqualityandsafetyforum.com. The website will also provide a forum where you can ask specific questions about your safety and medical quality improvement projects or mentor upcoming medical quality leaders.

References

1. Sackett DL, Rosenberg WM, Gray JA, Haynes RB, Richardson WS. Evidence based medicine: what it is and what it isn't. BMJ. 1996;312(7023):71–2.

Basic Principles of Consuming Academic Literature

Zaza Atanelov

Tools
AMSTAR, CONSORT, PRISMA, STROBE, Types of research studies, translational, clinical, quality improvement, primary, secondary, "bench research," review article, meta-analysis, guidelines, decision analysis, experimental vs observational, randomized controlled study, bias, blinding, intervention vs control, placebo, association, case report, case-controlled study, exposure, odds ratio, cohort study, incidence rate, cross-sectional study, survey, prospective vs retrospective, confounding, IMRAD format, null hypothesis, prognosis, screening, diagnosis, causation

Z. Atanelov (✉)
School of Medicine, New York Medical College,
Class of 2017-40 Sunshine Cottage Road,
Vahalla, NY 10595, USA

School of Health Sciences and Practice,
New York Medical College, Class of 2017-30 Plaza W,
Vahalla, NY 10595, USA
e-mail: zatanelov@gmail.com

L. Atanelov (ed.), *Resident's Handbook of Medical Quality and Safety*, DOI 10.1007/978-3-319-24190-6_21

- **Situation**: As clinicians we are responsible to drive our practice based on evidence published in academic literature [1].
- **Background**: Evidence-based medicine is currently taught as part of medical school curriculum [2].
- **Assessment:** Few clinicians, and even fewer medical students, are skilled in analyzing, understanding and implementing medical evidence into practice [3].
- **Recommendation**: Since a large part of medical safety and quality improvement work is based on aligning medical practice with current evidence, it is of utmost importance to develop, at least, a rudimentary systematic approach to understanding academic literature..

Please Note

This is just an *introductory chapter* on the basic principles to be aware of; we recommend reviewing the links provided by the *British Medical Journal* (http://www.bmj.com/about-bmj/resources-readers/publications/how-read-paper) for a more complete coverage of this topic.

Types of Clinical Studies

- **Laboratory vs. Informatics**
- **Clinical vs. Translational vs. Quality Improvement**

  - **Laboratory, "bench" or "basic" or "wet lab"** studies use artificial laboratory conditions to study **compounds, cells, or animals** to determine potential utility, efficacy, toxicity, and safety of interventions.

    Examples: Using a pipette to deliver an investigational anti-cancer compound to a rat model of a meningioma OR Analyzing the toxic effects of the same anti-cancer compound on the rat's bone marrow. These studies allow for lots of control of the environment and thereby minimize confounding (see below).
  - **Informatics** studies use computers to analyze biological or clinical information available as a hospital data set, as

an online data bank, or as part of the electronic medical record (EMR).

Example: Informatics can be used to analyze the compliance of nurses with twice/day tracking of patient vitals via patient EMR information. ***OR*** *Informatics can be used to mine data for mRNA splicing patterns via online data banks, like the human genome project.*

- **Clinical vs. Translational vs. Quality Improvement**
  - **Translational** studies are a subtype of clinical studies. They take successful laboratory studies and apply them to human subjects in order to "translate" the interventions with positive results, in the lab, in mice to positive results in people.
  - **Clinical** studies investigate human subjects and their associated medical and demographic information to investigate efficacy and safety of biological or behavioral interventions. Clinical studies generally allow for much less control of the environment compared to laboratory studies, but are more applicable to real life situations.

    Example: one can, as part of an experiment, feed a rat only carrots for 3 years to study the effects of carrots in causing cancer; however, a human subject normally would have a more varied diet, and observed cancer may not eve be a consequence of diet, but rather of a confounding factor like cigarette smoking.

  - **Quality Improvement (QI)** studies asses the extent of effort directed toward closing the gap between established medical guidelines and current practice in a hospital setting, for example.
- **Primary vs. Secondary Studies**
  - A "primary" research study starts with the original biopsychosocial-economical-clinical data, applies scientific methodology, and produces a set of results. Examples include case-control studies, randomized controlled studies, etc.

– A "secondary" research study analyzes and interprets results of primary studies.

- **Examples of secondary studies**:
  - **Review articles** summarize results of several studies on a particular topic; a **systemic review** will normally utilize rigorous methodology described in the article.

    Example: PubMed search of "aspirin" and "stroke" was utilized on May 30, 2013, to generate a list of articles that can be analyzed to include in a Review article that includes a comprehensive review of all the data.

  - **Meta-analyses** integrates numerical data from several primary studies.

    Example: Data from seven randomized controlled studies was combined to assess the overall effect of physical therapy vs. no physical therapy after total knee replacement.

  - **Guidelines** draw conclusions from prior studies/expert opinion on what and how to implement in medical practice.

    Example: Immediate surgical evaluation is indicated for patients with newly diagnosed cauda equina syndrome.

  - **Decision analyses** compare efficacy/safety of one set of clinical interventions in a particular order to another one.

    Example: Years of life-year gained for intervention A vs. B in brain cancer patients.

  - Online resources for secondary studies include:
    – Cochrane: http://www.cochrane.org/cochrane-reviews
    – Bandolier: http://www.jr2.ox.ac.uk/bandolier
    – BMJ: http://www.clinicalevidence.com
    – TRIP: http://www.tripdatabase.com

- **Experimental vs. Observational**
  - **Experimental Study**: An intervention (e.g., toxin, growth factor, cancer medicine) is applied to experimental subjects (e.g., lab rats, nerve cells, cancer patients) and the effects of the intervention are observed (e.g., lab rats die, nerve cells grow, cancer patients live longer) in order to understand the intervention's physiological effects and mechanism of action. Experimental studies seek to show **causation**.

    Example: This intervention/cancer medication successfully cured the cancer. One example of an experimental study is a Randomized Control Trial (RCT), which is a clinical experimental study. One of the goals of an RCT and other clinical experimental studies is to test and analyze interventions to correctly diagnose and treat illness.

- **What Goes into an Experimental Study?**
  - People are the subjects of clinical studies. They can be randomized, as is done in an **RCT**, or non-randomized. Randomization reduces and tries to eliminate selection/sampling **bias**.

    Example: Sampling bias due to non-random sampling of a target population (pregnant teenagers of low socioeconomic status) can cause the characteristics of the selected study population to differ from those of the target population. This may lead to results that may not be generalizable to the target population.

  - Interventions, like whether to take drug A, drug B or both, are controlled by the experimenters. However, sometimes you cannot control an intervention due to ethical reasons.

    Example: You are studying the risk of DVTs for your new estrogen analog in smokers vs. non-smokers. You cannot tell a people who don't smoke to start smoking and people who smoke to stop. Therefore, you end up with a non-randomized, non-controlled study.

- Studies can be triple blinded, where the investigators, study subjects and the researchers analyzing the data do not know who was in the intervention or in the non-intervention group. They can also be **double-blinded**, where just the investigators and subjects don't know who is in the intervention or non-intervention group. Additionally they can only be blinded to the subjects or not blinded at all. Blinding is utilized to reduce the influence of study subjects, researchers and doctors on the intervention and data analysis, which reduces bias.
  - **Intervention group** receives some type of intervention by the research team.
  - **Nonintervention group** may receive:
    - No intervention (to show efficacy)
    - Placebo (to show efficacy)
    - Alternative intervention (to show relative efficacy)

- **Observational Study:** Investigators observe experimental subjects (e.g., lab rats, nerve cells, cancer patients) and note/measure variable(s) of interest (e.g., affinity to particular types of food, life span, packs of cigarettes smoked a week). Observational studies normally show **association**

  Example: Smoking is associated with lung cancer. Examples of observational studies include case control, cohort, case reports/series, and cross-sectional/survey studies (see below). Observational clinical studies are often interested in etiology, harm, and prognosis of an illness.

- **Note: An association does not have to imply causation**. For instance, wearing a white coat at work is associated with **being** a physician, but wearing a white coat does not cause one to **become** a physician; on the other hand, smoking is both associated and has been shown to cause lung cancer.

Examples of Observational Studies

- **Case report** – describes a clinical experience with one patient; no particular research protocol is usually followed. Case series reports describe an experience with a small number of patients.

  Example: First report of drug X causing heart attack.

  – Usual use: New or rare diseases, adverse drug reactions.
  – Shortcoming: This particular clinical experience may not generalize to other patients with similar diagnosis.
  – Benefit: Quick to produce and low-cost efforts.

- **Case-control study** – outcome is measured before exposure. Examines a *set of exposures* in both **cases** (patients with illness) and **controls** (patients without illness) and assesses how the exposures differ between the two groups. Ideally, patients should **match** based on other possible confounders, e.g., age and sex. This is normally done retrospectively.

  Example: Male patients between ages of 60–65; ***case****, Guillain-Barre syndrome;* ***control****, no Guillain-Barre syndrome. Examine the many different exposures (cholesterol in diet, cigarette smoking, exercise, etc.) in both groups and assess if the amount of exposure is statistically different between the groups.*

  – Usual Use: Identify which **exposure(s)** is/are associated with the outcome in question, often used when cases are rare.
  – Shortcoming: Prone to selection and recall bias. Provides **odds ratio** (odds that the group with the outcome was exposed divided by the odds that people without the outcome were exposed), which approaches but does not always represent true relative risk of the exposure leading to the observed outcome. If prevalence of the studied disease is low the odds ratio approximates very close to relative risk.

- Benefit: Quick to produce, low-cost efforts, may need to enroll less patients and may obtain results purely on already available data.

- **Cohort study** – exposure is measured before the outcome. Groups patients by exposure (e.g., smoking vs. not) and examines the effect of the exposure on contributing to outcomes (e.g., stroke, cancer, heart attack).

  Example: People who smoked at least 40 packs of cigarettes a year are followed to assess their risk for developing cancer, stroke, and heart attack. The proportion(s) of outcome(s) in question is/are compared between the two groups.

  - Usual Use: Outcomes with high prevalence.
  - Shortcoming: Prone to attrition bias and change in methodology over time, expensive, takes long, need to enroll many patients.
  - Benefit: Produces true **incidence rate** (# of new cases divided by # of people at risk in a given time period) and **relative risk** (risk of an outcome in the exposed group divided by risk in the unexposed group).

- **Cross-sectional/survey** – measures prevalence of a particular variable within a particular short time segment.

  Example: Exit poll survey or prevalence of brain cancer in year 2014.

- **Prospective vs. Retrospective**

  - **Retrospective Study:** Analyzes events that took place in the past.

    Example: Starting with mothers who delivered children with fetal alcohol syndrome and asking them how much alcohol they drank during their pregnancy and how much folate they took. Retrospective studies can help identify what potential risk or protective factors are for a particular disease. ***Confounding and bias*** *(see below) are more common in these studies, and* *these studies provide weaker evidence than prospective studies but are faster and less costly to implement.*

- **Prospective Study:** Event of interest is expected to take place in the future.

  Example: A cancer medicine is administered to a group of patients and cancer remission in these patients is observed at 6 months after the intervention.

Sources of Error in Clinical Studies

- **Bias**
  - Error introduced during planning, implementing, and analyzing/publishing the study.
  - Types of bias and how to avoid it are described elsewhere [4].
  - See bias assessment tool for randomized clinical studies [5].
- **Confounding**
  - Variable(s) that was/were not accounted for but may impact results of the study unbeknownst to the investigator and lead to false conclusions. Confounding is a type of bias.

Intuitive Systematic Method to Analyze Studies (Adapted from [6])

Question 1: Why was the study done, and what clinical question were the authors addressing?
Question 2: What type of study was done?
Question 3: Was this design appropriate to the research?

Note: Most articles follow the IMRaD format [7]: introduction, methods, results, and discussion/conclusion. This method of assessing studies mirrors the basic article structure.

Question 1: Why was the study done, and what clinical question were the authors addressing?

Article *Introduction*

- *Should provide a background to the subject and clearly illustrate the hypothesis in question*
- *Was the hypothetico-deductive method utilized?*
- *Was this study assessing something of clinical/scientific relevance?*
- *Is this study repeating what was already done by a different group?*

- Null hypothesis (Ho): x = y

  (a) The opposite of the proposed hypothesis

- Alternative hypothesis (Ha): x ≠ y
- "Hypothetico-deductive" approach

  (a) Attempts to disprove or reject the null hypothesis (Ho) which in turn proves or leaves open the opportunity for the proposed hypothesis (Ha) to be true.
  (b) **Rejecting Ho does not prove that Ha must be true, for there may also be another alternative hypothesis which was not even examined.**

  Example: Ha: Smoking causes cancer. Ho: Smoking does not cause cancer. Hypothetico-deductive approach will attempt to disprove the null hypothesis that "smoking does not cause cancer."

Hypothesis types:

- Intervention/therapy

  (a) Is clopidogrel + aspirin co-therapy superior to aspirin alone in preventing strokes? Ho: aspirin = clopidogrel + aspirin; Ha: aspirin ≠ clopidogrel + aspirin
  (b) In this case one would compare the rate of strokes in each treatment arm and assess if the difference is statistically significant.

Table 1 Illustrates the relationship between common hypothetical study approaches and the most commonly utilized and best study designs to analyze the respective hypotheses.

Hypothesis type	Possible appropriate study design
Therapy/ intervention	Double-blind RCT is best; cohort study provides less evidence. Bias and confounding should be assessed
Diagnosis	Cross-sectional study may be appropriate in evaluating test administered vs. gold standard. **Validity** and **reliability** of the test need to be questioned
Screening	Cross-sectional study may be appropriate. Ask if test generalizes to larger populations and if it detects presymptomatic stage disease
Prognosis	Prospective cohort study may be appropriate. Ask how exhaustively was the development of complications assessed and how long was the cohort followed
Possible causation	RCT and prospective cohort studies are best for common problems, case controls for rare diseases, and case reports for initial findings raising the concern for causation

Table 2 Illustrates the relationship between different study designs and the most appropriate criteria to utilize in the analysis of the proposed study data.

Type of study	Guideline/criteria
Meta-analysis, review article	AMSTAR [8], PRISMA [9]
RCT	CONSORT [10]
Observational study	STROBE [11]

- Prognosis
  (a) What is the life expectancy of stage II small cell lung carcinoma patients?
- Causation
  (a) Does smoking cause cancer?
  (b) This is an example of a hypothesis test involving **dichotomous data**, which means the answer is either a yes or a no. In this case one would look at the prevalence (p1) of cancer in smokers and the prevalence (p2) of cancer in nonsmokers. Ho: $p1 = p2$; Ha: $p1 > p2$.
- Diagnosis
  (a) Can HbA1c be used to diagnose diabetes?
  (b) This is also an example of a hypothesis test involving dichotomous data. In this case one should look at the prevalence (p1) of diabetes in people with increased HbA1c levels and the prevalence (p2) of diabetes in people with normal or moderate HbA1c levels. Ho: $p1 = p2$; Ha: $p1 > p2$.
- Screening
  (a) How sensitive is the question "Do you still enjoy the things you used to enjoy?" to detect depression?
  (b) In this example, one would assess a group of patients suspected to have depression using this question alone (assigning a proportion p1 patients into "depressed" category) and compare it to the proportion (say p2) based on the **gold standard** definition of depression via the Diagnostic and Statistical Manual of Mental Disorders.

Question 2: What type of study was done?

Check the *Methods* section to identify the type of study design.

- Laboratory vs. Informatics
- Translational vs. Clinical vs. Quality Improvement

- Primary vs. secondary
- Observational vs. experimental etc.

Question 3: Was this design appropriate to the research hypothesis?

Check article *Discussion/Conclusion* sections.

Did the study meet the goals?

Did it disprove the null hypothesis (*Ho*)*?*

(Table 1)

Assess the level of evidence [adapted from http://www.cebm.net]Systemicreview/meta-analysis > RCT > cohort > case control > case report.

Use study assessment tools to further analyze the studies.

(Table 2)

If you have any questions about the information covered in this chapter or other medical safety and quality improvement-related topics, please contact us at http://www.medicalqualityandsafetyforum.com. The website will also provide a forum where you can ask specific questions about your safety and medical quality improvement projects or mentor upcoming medical quality leaders.

References

1. Dawes M, Summerskill W, Glasziou P, et al. Second international conference of evidence-based health care teachers and developers. Sicily statement on evidence-based practice. BMC Med Educ. 2005;5:1.
2. Bloch RM, Swanson MS, Hannis MD. An extended evidence-based medicine curriculum for medical students. Acad Med. 1997;72:431–2.
3. van Dijk N, Hooft L, Wieringa-de Waard M. What are the barriers to residents' practicing evidence-based medicine? A systematic review. Acad Med. 2010;85:1163–70.
4. Pannucci C, Wilkins E. Identifying and avoiding bias in research. Plast Reconstr Surg. 2010;126(2):619–25.

5. Higgins J, Altman D, et al. The cochrane collaboration's tool for assessing risk of bias in randomised trials. BMJ. 2011;343:d5928s.
6. Greenhalgh T. How to read a paper: getting your bearings (deciding what the paper is about). BMJ. 1997;315:243.
7. Luciana B, Periera S, Periera M. The introduction, methods, results, and discussion (IMRAD) structure: a fifty-year survey. J Med Libr Assoc. 2004;92(3):364–71.
8. Shea BJ, et al. Development of AMSTAR: a measurement tool to assess the methodological quality of systematic reviews. BMC Med Res Methodol. 2007;7:10.
9. Moher D, et al. Preferred reporting items for systematic reviews and meta-analyses: the PRISMA statement. BMJ. 2009;339:b2535.
10. Begg C, et al. Improving the quality of reporting of randomized controlled trials: the CONSORT statement. JAMA. 1996;276:6379.
11. von Elm E, et al. The Strengthening the Reporting of Observational Studies in Epidemiology (STROBE) statement: guidelines for reporting observational studies. Ann Intern Med. 2007;147(8):573–7.

Part V
Implementing Quality Improvement Interventions

Generating Creative Ideas as a Group for Quality Improvement

Sharon H. Kim

> **Tools**
> Idea generation, barriers, groupthink, hesitation, DMAIC, brainstorming

What

- Social science researchers have long documented the numerous challenges of maximizing creativity in both individuals and in groups [1].
- There are two phases of group creativity during which many of these challenges may materialize: (1) idea generation (suggesting ideas during brainstorming) and (2) idea selection (evaluating and selecting among suggested ideas).
- Stunted idea generation and/or subpar idea selection processes may inhibit the potential innovation and quality of quality improvement (QI) project outcomes.

S.H. Kim (✉)
Carey Business School and Armstrong Institute for Patient Safety and Quality, Johns Hopkins University, 100 International Drive, Baltimore, MD 21202, USA
e-mail: sharon.kim@jhu.edu

L. Atanelov (ed.), *Resident's Handbook of Medical Quality and Safety*, DOI 10.1007/978-3-319-24190-6_22

- Common Barriers to Idea Generation
  - Groupthink is a "psychological drive for consensus that suppresses dissent and appraisal of alternatives in cohesive decision-making groups" [2].
  - Hesitation to express ideas due to the fear that they might be judged harshly by peers and/or higher status members.
  - Social loafing or free riding that occurs when individuals in a group do not contribute to the discussion equitably.
  - The idea generation process becomes routinized (e.g., one member establishes him-/herself as the "thought leader" and routinely dominates the conversation).
  - Demographic and individual differences that come into play in terms of willingness to participate, social influence, and ability to persuade others (e.g., introversion/extraversion, gender, narcissism, national culture, etc.) [3].
- Common Barriers to Idea Selection
  - Hesitation to support an idea that does not already have support (i.e., challenges of expressing a dissenting or minority opinion).
  - Hesitation to reject or criticize an idea that is supported by a high-status member of the team.
  - Individual differences may influence the way ideas are perceived in terms of quality:
- For instance, extraverted individuals may be more adept at selling their ideas and influencing the group, while introverted individuals may find it difficult to pitch their ideas convincingly in a group setting.
- Recent research shows that narcissists are more effective at convincing others that their ideas are more creative even when those ideas are not superior to the ideas of others [4].
  - The idea selection process becomes routinized such that ideas are not fully vetted.
- For instance, some research has shown that in a typical four-person group, two people do 62 % of the talking [5]. In such cases, it is easy to see how idea selection may not be subject to critical thinking or rigorous review.

How

- Awareness of these challenges (see above) can be an important first step in facilitating creativity in QI groups and teams.
- Encourage open and active participation of all members of the team regardless of status, position, tenure, etc.
  - Research shows that when a group is exposed to minority (versus majority) opinions or dissent, that group is more likely to be creative [6, 7].
- When expressed, such opinions help the group think more divergently (versus convergently) which, in turn, may result in a more creative final outcome.
- Discourage or take steps to avoid routinized approaches to idea generation and selection.
- Take into consideration the composition of the team and design exercises and interventions to maximize creativity accordingly.
  - For example, if there is an overwhelming majority that is represented, take note to encourage the participation of other minority members.

Systematic Approach to Improving Creative Idea Generation and Selection Process in Groups Using DMAIC

Define

- Problem: Overcoming common barriers to group QI creativity
- Goal: Increasing creativity of QI idea generation and idea selection sessions
- Benefit: Improve probability of implementing higher quality QI solutions
- Scope: All QI groups and teams responsible for creative problem solving

Measure

- Identify potential barriers to QI idea generation and idea selection in groups.
- Formal, systematic tools to assess such barriers do not currently exist; however, these issues are so common that it can be assumed that there is ample room to improve in this domain (see suggestions above to identify potential barriers).
- Evaluate quality of idea generation and selection both pre- and post-intervention.
  - Please see below (under *Analyze*) for methods of assessing the quality of ideas generated.
- Consider measuring the following variables:
  - The number of ideas suggested per individual.
  - Total number of ideas suggested by the entire team.
  - Ask objective third-party individuals familiar with QI to evaluate the quality of the final, selected idea or ideas (anonymized data) by rating them for originality, appropriateness, and feasibility.
  - Monitor team members' engagement during sessions.
  - Survey team members to gauge satisfaction with the process.
- Note: any surveys should be conducted anonymously and carefully designed to promote constructive criticism and open sharing of ideas.
- Continue to identify additional opportunities for improvement and innovation in the idea generation and idea selection processes.

Analyze

- Conduct qualitative analyses of QI brainstorming and idea generation sessions to determine efficacy of teams and interventions.

- Identify and prioritize potential causes of the problem.
- Assess the magnitude of contribution of each cause to a quantitative marker of high-quality idea generation and selection.

Improve

- Depending on the makeup of QI groups and teams as well as additional identified barriers to creativity, teams may need to experiment with various interventions in order to figure out what works best for them.
- Suggestions for interventions to improve the quality of idea generation:
  - Randomize the order in which team members speak during brainstorming and idea generation sessions. This can prevent the same individuals from speaking most often or in the same order.
  - Collect some ideas anonymously and/or in advance. Consider spending some time at the beginning of the session going over them to get the group started down the right path.
  - Leaders may wish to make a habit of speaking last to allow others to contribute their ideas under less conformity pressure.
  - Set a very short time limit for brainstorming and encourage individuals to write down every idea regardless of feasibility. This can help reduce the pressure of sharing only those ideas that are considered to be "good."
  - Consider inviting individuals from affiliated QI teams to sit in from time to time to introduce new influences and sources of inspiration.
- Suggestions for interventions to improve the quality of idea selection:
  - Randomize the order in which individuals present constructive feedback of short-listed ideas.
  - Ask members to submit constructive critiques of short-listed ideas anonymously.

- If possible, consider leaving a break between the discussion of options and the final idea selection. This allows for ideas to incubate and reduces some of the psychological influences that may be affecting the perceived quality of options on the table.
- Leaders may wish to hold their opinions until the very end to encourage the full participation of other members during the selection process.
- Randomly select an individual to play the role of "devil's advocate." This person's duty is to be the voice of dissent in the idea selection process [8].

Control

- Select a particular set of variables that will be monitored after the *Improve* phase is complete to ensure that the gains of the intervention are sustained.

Potential Challenges

- Maintaining an environment that promotes group creativity requires a commitment to remain flexible. This can be especially difficult for busy QI groups and teams who may find it easier to repeat the same procedure every time for the sake of convenience.
- It may take some time to undo the existing habits and traditions of individual QI members and teams that may currently impede creative contributions.

Potential Successes

- Increasing the chances of identifying and implementing creative solutions to QI problems.
- Maximizing the creative QI potential of individual members as well as that of the collective.

- Encouraging the participation of all members helps increase creativity but also serves as a form of succession planning. By encouraging newer members to perform in this manner, these members can continue expressing their creativity as they continue to progress within the organization.
- Depending on how interventions are implemented, QI team members may be more intrinsically motivated to contribute in meetings.

Future Directions

The tools to solve these issues should be developed to meet the specific needs and characteristics of each QI team. In the development of such tools, consider taking advantage of the following helpful resources:

- **Empirical research in organizational behavior and social psychology:** Currently, there is great interest on the topic of creativity in organizations. QI teams may wish to capitalize on high-quality empirical studies to stay up to date on the latest findings and potentially helpful interventions.
- **Technological applications:** QI groups and teams may wish to investigate organizational and technological tools (e.g., survey tools, anonymous voting applications, planning and communication applications, etc.) to help make idea generation and selection more effective and efficient.

If you have any questions about the information covered in this chapter or other medical safety and quality improvement-related topics, please contact us at http://www.medicalqualityandsafetyforum.com. The website will also provide a forum where you can ask specific questions about your safety and medical quality improvement projects or mentor upcoming medical quality leaders.

References

1. Amabile TM. Creativity in context: update to the social psychology of creativity. Boulder: Westview Press; 1996.
2. Janis IL. Victims of groupthink: a psychological study of foreign-policy decisions and fiascoes. Oxford, UK: Houghton Mifflin; 1972.
3. Goncalo JA, Flynn FJ, Kim SH. Are two narcissists better than one? The link between narcissism, perceived creativity, and creative performance. Pers Soc Psychol Bull. 2010;36(11):1484–95.
4. Goncalo JA, Kim SH. Distributive justice beliefs and group idea generation: does a belief in equity facilitate productivity? J Exp Soc Psychol. 2010;46(5):836–40.
5. Thompson L. Fortune magazine: how to neutralize a meeting tyrant. 2013. http://fortune.com/2013/02/11/how-to-neutralize-a-meeting-tyrant/. Accessed 7 July 2014.
6. Nemeth CJ. Differential contributions of majority and minority influence. Psychol Rev. 1986;93(1):23.
7. Nemeth CJ, Staw BM. The tradeoffs of social control and innovation within groups and organizations. In: Berkowitz L, editor. Advances in experimental social psychology, vol. 22. New York: Academic; 1989. p. 175–210.
8. Nemeth C, Brown K, Rogers J. Devil's advocate versus authentic dissent: Stimulating quantity and quality. Eur J Soc Psychol. 2001;31(6):707–20.

Scope

Kevin C. Platt

Tools
Project charter, Project Scope Guide

Once you select the process targeted for improvement, it is critical to determine optimal parameters to successfully achieve the desired goal. Just as a good photographer chooses the correct lens and then aims the camera skillfully to compose a perfect shot, the quality improvement champion must ensure the appropriate parts of a process are defined clearly by the scope. Henri Cartier-Bresson, the famous French photographer considered to be the father of photojournalism, was opposed to cropping photographs or otherwise manipulating his images in any way in the darkroom [1]. He insisted on getting it right during framing and composition. This same discipline will lead to better results and clearer presentation in quality improvement work.

K.C. Platt (✉)
Department of Inpatient Rehabilitation,
MedStar Good Samaritan Hospital,
5601 Loch Raven Boulevard, Baltimore, MD 21239, USA
e-mail: kevin.c.platt@medstar.net

L. Atanelov (ed.), *Resident's Handbook of Medical Quality and Safety*, DOI 10.1007/978-3-319-24190-6_23

When preparing the project charter during the *Define* phase, take time to compose your plan correctly by determining the beginning and end points for a variety of parameters. The deliverable for this stage is a clear understanding of what is *in scope* (included in project) and what is *out of scope* (excluded from project) which will inform the data collection and measurement, analysis, improvement, and ultimately control of the process. When team members agree on what items are in scope, they communicate to all involved what the project will focus on, while deeming items out of scope is a way to keep the project to a size that is manageable, so that it may be completed within a short time frame [2]. Table 1 provides examples of several parameters to consider when designing your QI project.

Once a variable is selected to be measured, it must be defined objectively and in as much detail as possible, based on the acceptable error for that variable. For example, if length of stay (LOS) is defined in your project as date of discharge minus date of admission, and days is the unit of measure, you will have to accept that observations with LOS = 1 day can have actual hospital stays ranging in duration from less than 1 h (e.g., admit January 1st at 11:45 PM; discharge January 2nd 12:15 AM), to the full 24 h.

The term "project scope creep" refers to the tendency of a project to grow in its scope, often without the availability of additional time, resources, expertise, or information required to get it done. The breadth and depth of a project can also be detrimentally whittled down to the point where it becomes ineffective, unsuccessful, or irrelevant, if the project champion does not scope the project aggressively enough to affect meaningful and lasting improvement in quality. A project with a scope that is either too broad or too narrow will be difficult to complete successfully.

Table 1 Project Scope Guide

Parameter	Scope question	Sample "in scope"	Sample "out of scope"
Degree	What is the severity threshold of the medical condition or problem you are trying to improve?	Stage III pressure ulcers; Registration wait times of 20–30 min	Pressure ulcers less than or greater than Stage III; Registration wait times less than 20 min or greater than 30 min
Demographics	What are the patient characteristics that define where improvement is necessary?	Rate of hospital readmission within 30 days for patients who live alone in the community	Readmission rates for patients who live with family, in an institution, or in an aggregate living situation
Diagnosis	Which specific conditions are you focusing on?	Patients with acute CVA and right upper extremity hemiplegia	Patients with acute CVA and left hemiplegia, or no hemiplegia of the upper extremity
Payor	Is there variation in the process related to how the health care is funded?	Length of stay for patients with Medicaid as the primary insurance	Length of stay for patients with insurance other than Medicaid; patients for whom Medicaid eligibility status has not yet been determined
Person	Whose behavior am I attempting to change?	Emergency department physicians assigned on night shift	All physician assistants and ED physicians assigned on day shift

(continued)

Table I (continued)

Parameter	Scope question	Sample "in scope"	Sample "out of scope"
Place	Where does the activity take place?	Acute care patients treated on the 5th Floor Oncology Unit	Acute care patients who are transferred from the 5th Floor Oncology Unit to another unit, prior to discharge
Procedure	Which part of the overall process do I want to impact?	Use of the computerized physician order entry (CPOE) order set for M-W-F routine lab orders	All lab orders other than M-W-F routine labs
Program	What is the operational structure around this process?	Patients who are admitted to the hospital for acute medical services	Patients who are in the hospital under observation status
Protocol	Which intervention(s) is/are being studied?	Clinical appropriateness of central line placements performed by the surgeon on duty	Rate of central line associated blood stream infections (CLABSI)
Time	What is the target date/period for the change to take place?	In the final quarter of the current reporting year	Cases discharged prior to October 1st

For example, a project initially designed to address unnecessary laboratory tests for patients in an inpatient rehabilitation specialty unit might become too difficult to manage if it is broadened to include the medical-surgical areas of the hospital. Consider that rehabilitation patients in the example are managed by a group of physical medicine and rehabilitation physicians, residents, and physician assistants with whom you have been working closely, while patients on the medical-surgical units are attended to by hospitalists, other residents, and hundreds of community physicians. On the other hand, if the same project is aimed at only one of two nearly identical rehabilitation units that are part of the same program, the improvement on the pilot unit might be less than what could be achieved if all personnel (both units) were focused simultaneously on the same QI project. While the intent may have been to make the work more manageable by excluding one of the units, having different expectations and procedures based on a patient's location might lead to less overall compliance on the focus unit.

Project scope may be too broad if:

- Unable to produce concise, focused charter
- Difficult to identify sources for essential data
- Not enough time and/or resources to collect and analyze data
- Project team size too large (ideal 6–8 individuals)
- Difficult to explain desired outcome

Project scope may be too narrow if:

- Out-of-scope items seem more urgent than in-scope items
- Out-of-scope items are easily incorporated into project
- Project involves too few stakeholders
- Lack of enthusiasm among stakeholders
- Improvement unlikely to "stick" within existing culture and framework

Get to Know the Informatics Team

The electronic medical record (EMR) is a repository for an increasing amount of clinical information. As hospitals continue to adopt EMR and expand their use of electronic documentation, more and more information is becoming available to researchers and those doing quality improvement work. Getting information out of these complex systems is not always as easy as entering it, however. Consulting with an informatics professional about your project concept is a great way to learn about what data is available and can help you determine the optimal scope boundaries.

List of Terms Used

Scope	The boundaries for a QI project, including in scope (included) and out of scope (excluded)
In scope	Included in the project
Out of scope	Excluded from the project
Project charter	The document that defines the project problem, goals, expected benefits, scope, and other details
Project scope creep	Tendency of a project to grow in its scope, often without the availability of additional time, resources, expertise, or information required to get it done
Informatics team	Professionals who are trained in both clinical and technical aspects of the electronic medical record (EMR), including how to extract meaningful data for use in QI and research

If you have any questions about the information covered in this chapter or other medical safety and quality improvement-related topics, please contact us at http://www.medicalqualityandsafetyforum.com. The website will also provide a forum where you can ask specific questions about your safety and medical quality improvement projects or mentor upcoming medical quality leaders.

References

1. Kim E. 10 Things Henri Cartier-Bresson can teach you about street photography. Eric Kim Photography Blog [web log]. 2011. Retrieved Oct 2014, from http://erickimphotography.com/blog/2011/08/22/10-things-henri-cartier-bresson-can-teach-you-about-street-photography/
2. DeFeo JA, Swayne B, editors. Juran Lean Six Sigma Yellow Belt for Healthcare. Juran Institute; 2013. Southington, CT

How to Select and Scope a Project

Laura Winner and Richard Hill

Tools
Goal tree, Project charter, Scoping worksheet

You'll likely encounter many opportunities to improve patient care delivery processes on a daily basis. In this chapter, we will share the best practices for selecting the "right" project and scope in order to improve your likelihood of success.

Project Selection

Choose a Project That

- **Aligns to strategic aims**
  - Your project will compete for scarce resources to support data collection and interventions. Linking with strategic aims will increase your likelihood for access to those scarce resources.

L. Winner (✉) • R. Hill
Armstrong Institute for Patient Safety and Quality, Johns Hopkins Medicine, 750 E. Pratt St, Baltimore, MD 21202, USA
e-mail: lwinner@jhmi.edu

L. Atanelov (ed.), *Resident's Handbook of Medical Quality and Safety*, DOI 10.1007/978-3-319-24190-6_24

- A goal tree can help map the improvement project you are considering to the strategic aims of the organization. In the example below, two pressing quality and safety issues are represented: surgical site infection and deep vein thrombosis/pulmonary embolism (DVT/PE) prevention.

See Fig. 1.

- **Links with existing efforts when possible**
- Publicly reported measures have grown exponentially and most healthcare organizations have a cadre of quality improvement specialists working to measure and improve performance to these metrics. Partnering with these teams can smooth your path to improvement.
- **Has stakeholder support**
- A common pitfall of projects is a lack of key stakeholder buy-in and support. Stakeholders likely have other pressing priorities that may prevent them from fully supporting the initiative at a particular time, such as the launch of a new EMR, opening of a new building, Joint Commission visit pending, etc. Understanding stakeholder level of support for the project helps identify potential barriers and design effective strategies to overcome those barriers [1].

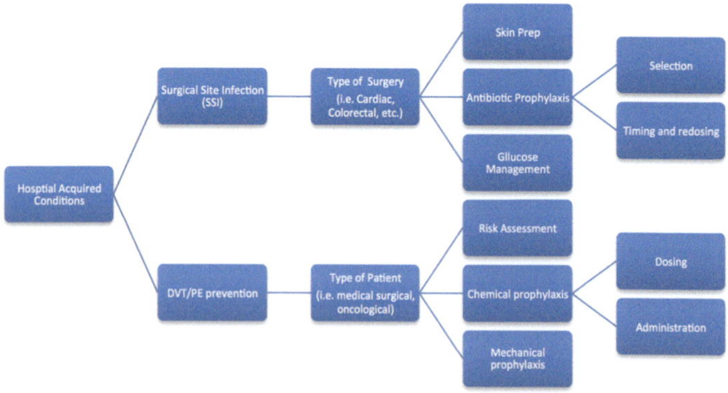

FIG. 1 Goal tree-aligning large-scale strategic goals to smaller scoped tactical projects

It can also inform scope by identifying areas with the greatest stakeholder support and higher likelihood for success.

- **Can be accomplished in a reasonable time frame**

Consider people's time to devote to the project as well as access to the necessary data to identify interventions and measure progress toward goal. Sufficient time should be built into the project to establish sustainability of results.

Once you have selected a project, it is time to draft your project charter. This tool will assist you in providing additional definition and clarity necessary to obtain approval and buy-in.

Project Charter

Description

A tool that summarizes key project information

Purpose

Provides a concise, detailed summary of the who, what, where, when, and how of your project in order to align all stakeholders, reduce ambiguity, and help prevent scope creep

Key Points

- Developed in concert with the project champion (sponsor)
- Dynamic – Changes over time to reflect project progression. Used as a team "touchstone" to keep everyone focused on the goal
- Changes must be vetted with the project champion.

Example

See Fig. 2.

Project Name: Blood Wastage Reduction	Champion: E. Smith, MD
Team Leader: D. Johnson	**Project Mentor:** S. Robinson, MBB
Problem Statement: Approximately 4.4% of our blood issued from, and returned to the blood bank is wasted. Loss of this precious resource results in patient safety issues and staff dissatisfaction.	**Project Goal:** Reduce the baseline rate of blood wastage from 4.4% to 2% (or less) by February 2015
Key Metric (Y): % of blood wasted = Units of blood returned to BB unused w/temp>10C / Total units issued from the BB	**Scope:** Limited to red blood cell units (RBCs) issued to and returned from the operating rooms, excludes units wasted as a result of the tube system.
Team Members: S. Ringley, RN L. McBurney, PA-C C. Hill – Blood Bank Tech B. Falk, MD	**Benefits:** Improved staff satisfaction, reduced cost through purchase of fewer red blood cell units – est. $200K/yr.
	Timeline: Define - Aug. 2014, Measure – Oct. 2014, Analyze - Nov. 2014, Improve -Dec. 2015, Control -Feb. 2015

FIG. 2 Example of a project charter describing a blood waste reduction initiative

Project Charter Components

Problem Statement

Description

A brief, compelling characterization of the current state and the need for the project

Purpose

Provides a common, relatable understanding of the problem and a need for stakeholder involvement

Key Points

- Includes the "burning platform" – compelling language to prompt people to join your team
  - Should answer the question of "So what?" or "Why should I care?"

- Components – *the current condition* results in (or leads to) *something undesirable* (burning platform)
- Includes specific data (if available)

Example (Poorly Defined)

- Our blood waste is too high.

Example (Improved)

- Approximately 4.4 % of our blood issued from and returned to the blood bank is wasted. Loss of this precious resource results in patient safety issues and staff dissatisfaction.

Key Metric aka Project Y or "Big Y"

Description

A *single* measurement of project success

Purpose

Tracks progress toward the goal.

Key Points

- List only *one* metric and explain the calculation, e.g., measurement = numerator/denominator.
- Must be a meaningful measure of the problem and goal
- The data must be attainable and be obtainable on a frequent basis – daily, weekly, and monthly.
- Simple is better! Avoid complexity in your measure.

Example (Poorly Defined)

- % of blood wasted.

Example (Improved)

- % of blood wasted = units of blood returned to BB unused w/temp >10 C/total units issued from the BB.

Goal

Description

Brief statement of desired future state vs. baseline in measurable terms

Purpose

Defines project success

Key Points

- List only *one* overarching goal that will determine success (multiple goals create confusion).
- Should include verbs such as increase, decrease, and improve
- Components – *Improve*/increase/decrease *the metric* from *baseline measure* to *improved target measure* by *a point in time*
- Your goal should be SMART – *S*pecific, *M*easurable, *A*ttainable, *R*esults oriented, *T*ime bound (adapted from Doran's original criteria of specific, measurable, assignable, realistic, and time related) [2].

Example (Poorly Defined)

- Reduce blood waste from current levels.

Example (Improved)

- Reduce the baseline rate of blood wastage from 4.4 % to 2 % (or less) by February 2015.

Scope Statement

Description

A definition of your project's boundaries

Purpose

Provides clarification of what data and factors will be included and those that will be specifically excluded from your project (more detail to follow in the Project Scope section)

Key Points

- Helps prevent scope creep (results in a protracted project length)
- Use key words such as "includes", "excludes" and "limited to" to clearly communicate project boundaries.
- Consider listing specific departments, locations, and process steps to limit the size of your project.
- List parameters such as "must be done at no cost," "no increases to staff or budget", etc.

Example (Poorly Defined)

- Red blood cells only.

Example (Improved)

- Limited to red blood cell units (RBCs) issued to and returned from the operating rooms, excludes units wasted as a result of the tube system

Benefit

Description

Anticipated/realized favorable outcomes (excluding the goal) attained through the project

Purpose

Provides justification for doing the project in addition to the direct benefit of achieving the project goal

Key Points

- List any hard benefits – cost reduction or revenue increase that can be assigned a dollar amount
- List any soft benefits – things known to be good but difficult to quantify in terms of dollars
- List any cost avoidance – budgeted unspent costs that will not be realized due to the project
- Review any estimated hard or cost avoidance benefits with finance to ensure accuracy. Convert dollar estimates to actual numbers (when known).

Example (Poorly Defined)

- Improved staff morale

Example (Improved)

- Improved staff satisfaction, reduced cost through purchase of fewer red blood cell units – est. $200 K/year

Team Members

Description

A listing by name and role for each member participating in the project

Purpose

Communicates involvement, ownership, recognition, and accountability

Key Points

- Your role is project leader (list in charter heading section).
- Limit to 12 members or less – use credentials for role description only, e.g., MD, RN.
- Composition should be mostly frontline (those actually doing the work).
- Use ad hoc members if not needed at every meeting, e.g., finance, IT.
- Include a champion (sponsor) – high-level person to mentor and remove barriers.
- Include other mentor resources such as Black Belts or other project management experts

Example (Poorly Defined)

- Sarah Ringley, Lindsay McBurney, Caitlyn Hill

Example (Improved)

- Sarah Ringley, RN; Lindsay McBurney, PA-C; Caitlyn Hill, Blood Bank Tech.

Timeline

Description

A projected duration of the project by phase from start through completion

Purpose

Establishes stakeholder time commitment expectations.

Key Points

- Convey dates by each framework phase used – PDSA, DMAIC, etc.
- Revisit frequently and modify based on new information or actual phase completion.

Ensure sufficient time is factored in the "Improve phase" to demonstrate sustainability of results

Example (Poorly Defined)

- Estimated Project Completion – Feb. 2015

Example (Improved)

- Define – Aug. 2014, Measure – Oct. 2014, Analyze – Nov. 2014, – Dec. 2015, Control – Feb. 2015

Project Scope

Just as physicians must assimilate a large amount of anecdotal and hard data to zero in on and treat the cause of a patient's illness, quality improvement project leaders must assimilate a large amount of anecdotal and objective data to effectively scope quality improvement projects [3]. To do this well, you need to decide with your champion and team what is "in scope" and "out of scope." As David Garrett points out in his book *Project Pain Reliever*, it is important to establish your "project perimeter" [4] through the creation of a scope document that clearly lists not only what you *will do* but just as importantly what you *will not do.*

Questions that can assist you with rightsizing your project scope are listed in Table 1.

TABLE 1 Project scoping worksheet

Problem to be addressed (per the project charter): What is the problem you are targeting? What improvement are you hoping to achieve? How will you measure this?
Patient population: Which patient populations will be included/excluded? *(Will the focus be the inpatient or outpatient setting or both? Will this be hospital wide or department/service/unit specific? Will the focus be on adults, pediatrics, or both? Any other important exclusions?)*
Process steps: Which process steps will be included? *(Will the project focus on the entire process or a subset of the process,* *i.e., arrival to the ED through the decision to admit?)*

Tips to Effective Project Scoping

Tip #1: Engage Your Project Sponsor and Stakeholders Early to Rightsize the Scope for Your Project

(Stakeholders include the project sponsor or any group of people who may be affected by the project. A helpful Lean Sigma tool to identify a stakeholder of the process is the SIPOC diagram.)

SIPOC

Description

A tool that is used to identify suppliers, inputs, process steps, outputs, and customers

Purpose

Provides an inclusive list of relevant project elements for improved understanding and analysis and reveals important stakeholders of the process

Key Points (Refer to Figs. 3 and 4)

- Begin by listing 4–8 *high-level* process steps – perform the following for each step:
  - Input column – list each thing the process step uses or requires
  - Output column – list the key things the process step produces
  - Supplier column – list each person/group of persons supplying the inputs to the process
  - Customer column – list each person/group of persons receiving outputs from the process step
- Suppliers and customers should be considered for team inclusion.
- Inputs are areas of focus where defects may occur.
- Outputs may be used as process measures.

Tip#2: Scope Your Project Within Your Sphere of Influence

While large-scale, cross-departmental projects are attractive, they typically consume large amounts of time, require immense political buy-in, and are generally reserved for veteran project managers. An effective strategy for medical interns and residents is to narrow the scope to a specific service, unit, or clinic for faster project completion with a higher likelihood of success.

Tip #3: Let Data Guide You to a Targeted Scope

It is common for the initial project scope to be larger than desired because data is not available to indicate key areas of

S	I	P	O	C
Suppliers	Inputs	Process (4-8 steps)	Outputs	Customers
The people or entities that provide INPUTS to the PROCESS	Things that the PROCESS requires to function normally	First Step Second Step Last Step	Things that the PROCESS produces	The people or entities that receive OUTPUTS from the PROCESS

FIG. 3 SIPOC diagram used to capture the suppliers, inputs processes, outputs, and customers of the process

S	I	P	O	C
Suppliers	Inputs	Process	Outputs	Customers
Provider, Nurse, Blood Supplier	Pt information Blood, Requisition	Blood is requested	Queue is created	Blood Bank Tech
Blood Bank Techs	Packaging, temp indicator, labels	Unit(s) prepped	Unit(s) packed/ ready for pick-up	Nurse, Tech
Nurse, Tech	Transport cart, Tube system	Unit(s) transported	Blood available at location for transfusion	Patient, Provider, Nurse
Nurse, Tech	Unit(s)	Unit(s) returned	Unit(s) in BB	Blood Bank Tech
Blood Bank Tech	Unit(s), Temp. Indicator, time out of BB	Unit(s) dispositioned	Determination - re-issue or waste	Blood Bank Tech

FIG. 4 SIPOC diagram applied to delivery of blood products to the operating

opportunity and focus. Simple analysis of data can provide the frequency and/or severity of issues by attribute, e.g., departments, services, units, etc. The scope may then be narrowed to address issues in specific areas that contribute most to the problem.

Tip #4: Guard Against Scope Creep

Despite your best efforts to clearly define the scope of your project, well-intended colleagues will ask to expand the project scope. This can lead to a drain of resources away from your main objective, increase the time to project completion, and may even cause the project to stall. The best defense against this is a well-documented project scope statement that clearly articulates to the team what is in and out of the scope. While not foolproof, this helps deter scope creep.

Let's walk through an example to illustrate the approach to defining project scope.

Example

A second year surgical resident on rotation in the surgical ICU of a large academic medical center was responsible for the care of an otherwise healthy young patient who developed the life-threatening complication of pulmonary embolism. As a result of this experience, the resident has become passionate about applying evidence-based practices to prevent avoidable DVT and PE. She mentions her interest to the residency director who recommends she attend the next Lean Sigma course to learn robust tools for improvement.

One of the requirements for participation in the course is to describe the project to which she will apply the Lean Sigma learning. Since this is new territory for her, she consults a Lean Sigma Master Black Belt to help her think through her project. The Master Black Belt, who is skilled in scoping quality improvement projects, walks her through the scoping worksheet (Table 2).

Table 2 Scoping worksheet

Problem to be addressed: **What is the problem you are targeting?** • *Prevent avoidable DVT/PE complications.* **What improvement are you hoping to achieve?** • *Improve the DVT risk assessment screening and ordering process.* **How will you measure this?** • *Percent of patients for whom the appropriate chemical and mechanical prophylaxis is ordered.*
Patient population: **Which patient populations will be included/excluded?** ***In scope (includes):*** *Adult surgical inpatients undergoing orthopedic surgery* • ***Out of scope (excludes):*** *Pediatric patients, ambulatory surgical outpatients, nonsurgical inpatients*
Process steps: **Which process steps will be included?** ***Includes:*** *Preoperative risk assessment and instructions, post-op risk assessment, and admission orders* • ***Excludes:*** Implementation of physician orders/patient refusal

Completing the scoping worksheet aids in refining the project scope

If you have any questions about the information covered in this chapter or other medical safety and quality improvement-related topics, please contact us at http://www.medicalqualityandsafetyforum.com. The website will also provide a forum where you can ask specific questions about your safety and medical quality improvement projects or mentor upcoming medical quality leaders.

References

1. Project Management Institute. A guide to the project management body of knowledge (PMBOK guide). 5th ed. Newtown Square: Project Management Institute; 2013.
2. Doran GT. There's a S.M.A.R.T. way to write management's goals and objectives. Manage Rev. 1981;70(11):35–6.
3. Lynch DP, Bertolino S, Cloutier E. How to scope DMAIC projects. Qual prog. 2003;36(1):37–41.
4. Garrett D. Project pain reliever: a just-in-time handbook for anyone managing projects. Ft. Lauderdale: J. Ross Pub; 2012.

Communication Tools in Healthcare: Basics

Solomon Rojhani and R. Samuel Mayer

Tools
SBAR, callout, checkback, handoff, sign-out, briefing, huddle, crew resource management, teach-back, Ask Me 3, SPIKES, team monitoring, cross-monitoring, IMSAFE, multidisciplinary rounds, red rules, team facilitation, two-challenge rule, CUS words, DESC script

S. Rojhani (✉)
Department of Physical Medicine and Rehabilitation, The Johns Hopkins University School of Medicine, 600 North Wolfe Street Phipps 160, Baltimore, MD 21287, USA
e-mail: srojhan1@jhmi.edu

R.S. Mayer
Department of Physical Medicine and Rehabilitation, The Johns Hopkins University School of Medicine, 600 Wolfe Street, Phipps #198, Baltimore, MD 21287, USA
e-mail: rmayer2@jhmi.edu

L. Atanelov (ed.), *Resident's Handbook of Medical Quality and Safety*, DOI 10.1007/978-3-319-24190-6_25

Communication

Adequate communication means clearly and accurately exchanging information among team members. Teamwork and communication gaps are very common in healthcare and represent a preventable cause of patient injury [1]:

(a) Developing effective communication:

  (i) Components of an effective team are those that provide a nurturing environment to foster effective teamwork and eventually lead to efficient communication. Many of these strategies have been defined above. Common barriers to effective communication among team members are listed below:

   1. Individual expectations
   2. Personality traits, difference, and cultural background
   3. Demographic differences including age, gender, etc.
   4. Established or imagined hierarchy
   5. Rivalry or conflicting professional identities
   6. Varying levels of education and qualifications
   7. Reward or punitive programs
   8. Differing levels of accountability and responsibility
   9. Complexity of care

  (ii) Determining personality types can often predict communication styles. This may range from passive to aggressive. An assertive middle-ground approach is often preferred in most situations [1, 2]:

   1. The passive individual often fails to express thoughts and opinions by attempting to appease and avoiding conflict at all costs. Persons may be sarcastic and give up with resentment. Passive individuals often remain silent.
   2. Aggressive individuals often intend to dominate and win. Thoughts are often self-centered and

expressions are commonly emotionally driven or based on feelings. These individuals may be seen as inappropriate and unprofessional based on their style of information delivery.

3. Assertiveness is a positive way or relaying information while remaining respectful of others. There is a value in all parties contributing. The individuals remain firm while stating "yes" when indicated and "no" when appropriate. This principle is applied appropriately when the common goal is appreciated, avoiding personalization, understanding patient-centered care, and placing safety first.

(b) Improving communication:

(i) Tools to improve communication have been extensively researched and adapted to clinical settings. These tools are often derived from military or aviation settings, which rely heavily on developing adequate communication in order to reduce errors in the workplace. Tools can be used to improve mutual support, communication, leadership, situation monitoring, listening skills, and both individual and group strategies [3, 4]:

1. SBAR – Developed initially by the military, SBAR is a structured communication tool used to effectively relay information. Commonly employed in briefing a team member in urgent situations, SBAR is especially useful when communicating across hierarchy lines. Often there may not be a recommendation although further evaluation or attention can be requested. Presented is a mock interaction between a nurse, using the SBAR technique, and a physician:

(i) Situation – What is going on with the patient?

1. Example: "Mr. X has a severe headache."

(ii) Background – What is the clinical scenario?

1. Example: "Mr. X had a bleed in his brain two weeks prior and has been feeling different all day. His blood pressure is significantly elevated."

(iii) Assessment – What do I think the problem is?

1. Example: "I am worried that he may be having another bleed."

(iv) Recommendation – What would I recommend?

1. Example: "Please come and assess the patient immediately."

2. Callout – Strategy to communicate critical information; informs all team members simultaneously during emergency situations and is often used in procedural settings. Callouts should utilize simple language spoken clearly and loudly. For instance, in the OR, a surgeon may state: "We will begin in 5 min" or "We will need to X-ray the spine in 10 min."
3. Checkback – Closed loop communication between a sender and a receiver; the sender initiates message → the receiver accepts message and provides feedback confirmation of receipt → the sender verifies message was received.
4. Handoff – A transfer of information and authority or responsibility during transitions of care. A sign-out is a common handoff tool used to transfer patient care among individuals or entities. "I PASS the BATON," an acronym for a lesser known tool, may also be useful in handoff situations:

(i) Sign-out essentials include the use of written and verbal media, minimization of distractions, preparation of report, and knowing sign-out details and patient plan. A face-to-face interaction is preferred. Sign-out reporting should be clear, concise, and as complete as possible.

(ii) Steps to perform an adequate sign-out include sharing clinical basics, providing a to-do list with alerts to any urgent actions, preparing cross coverage with "heads up" on anticipated concerns, and summarizing the report.

(iii) "I PASS the BATON" is an acronym that includes Introduction, Patient, Assessment, Situation, Safety, Background, Actions, Timing, Ownership, and Next. A sample telephone sign-out between two residents at different facilities has been provided below (Table 1).

5. Briefing – A discussion between two or more people, often between a team, and using succinct information pertinent to an upcoming event. A briefing maps out the plan of care and identifies daily goals by heightening awareness of the situation. Roles and responsibilities need to be identified at the onset. Briefings take place before the action has begun.
6. Team huddle – An event where team members come together to review patient data and decide on a course of action. A huddle can be prearranged like team meetings or as needed when a patient's condition requires a change in course of action. A key point is that anyone can call a team huddle at any point in time. Huddles differ from briefings in that huddles are created in developing situations and often deal with emerging information.
7. Active listening – A tool used to retain information and gain information by focusing on the information being presented and processing this information. The listener must be focused on the speaker and should be able to read back the information once delivered to the listener. It is crucial that the listener be able to maintain comfortable eye contact and body language. Responses should not be

Table 1 Demonstrates the "I PASS the BATON" method. This may be an effective tool during hand offs or signouts, , , where critical information is relayed

I	Introduction – identify the individuals involved	"I am resident Y from Oaks Medical Center calling to inform you about patient X"
P	Patient – identify the patient	"Patient X is a 23-year-old Caucasian male whom I am referring to your headache clinic"
A	Assessment – describe the chief complaint, vitals, and symptoms	"His chief complaint is one month of intermittent headaches located bilaterally at the temples, lasting wenty minutes at a time and occurring five to seven times a day. Pain is described in a band-like distribution, sometimes knifelike, and does not radiate. They are aggravated by stress and improve with rest. Associated symptoms include blurry vision"
S	Situation – describe the current circumstances, changes, and response to treatment	"Initially the headaches improved with over-the-counter medications. They have since worsened and have not been as responsive"
S	Safety concerns – critical findings and information	"He had an initial CT scan which was negative. Other laboratory workup was normal. He is allergic to dust and penicillin"
B	Background – medical history and medications	"Patient X denies previous hospitalizations or any comorbidities. He is not taking any medications"

A	Action – describe the actions taken	"Patient X had a negative CT scan and normal laboratory values during his visit to my clinic. I would like him to visit your clinic in addition to meeting with a therapist and beginning a headache log in order to better manage pain and stress"
T	Timing – mention the prioritization of events	"I believe that because of his stress level, he should be seen within a month"
O	Ownership – identify responsible parties	"I will continue to be the primary resident caring for this patient and I am requesting a consultation in your clinic"
N	Next – decide on a plan of care	"I am asking for you to see him within a month for management of his headaches and will send you all the pertinent information. He will then follow up with me and additional therapists"

framed while the speaker delivers the message. Listeners should confirm receipt of information by using additional confirmatory language such as: "I understand" or "Yes, I agree with you." This demonstrates to the speaker that his or her voice has been heard.

(ii) Crew resource management (CRM) and high-reliability organizations (HRO) [3–5]:

1. CRM was developed by experts in the field of aviation to improve team management and safety across the industry after understanding that 70% of flight accidents derived from communication failures.
2. Applying a CRM model to medicine includes:

   (i) Creation of a system that is capable of handling errors through redundancy, standardization, and checklists.
   (ii) Designing safe processes and procedures while avoiding placing blame. Ensure immunity and maintain a nonthreatening approach.
   (iii) Turning mistakes into learning opportunities by debriefing and establishing risk prevention programs.
   (iv) Establishing a program to identify risk, analyze, and break down lessons taught throughout the clinical community.

3. Commercial aviation and nuclear energy have been paradigms of high-reliability industries. Many initiatives have been implemented in order to translate the idea of a high-reliability organization to the medical field. Yet still, every year millions of individuals are adversely affected by preventable harm. An HRO strives toward the ultimate goal of decreasing accidents by creating a culture of safety and awareness. Highlighted below are five hallmark principles of HROs. Investigators have subsequently developed different frameworks and

described numerous examples of successful patterns reflected in the activity of such HROs.

4. Five principles of HRO include:

   (i) Preoccupation with failure – individuals within the system should be constantly searching for ways to prevent accidents and failure.
   (ii) Avoiding oversimplification of environmental factors – safety concerns may present themselves in many different ways and vigilance is crucial.
   (iii) Sensitivity to operations – the smallest changes in performance should be noted as this may have profound influence throughout the system.
   (iv) Commitment to resilience – when errors do occur, they are quickly contained and managed so as not to have disabling effects at any point in time.
   (v) Deference to expertise – decision-making should often remain in the hands of those who are most apt at dealing with the problem.

(iii) Improving communication between healthcare workers and patients:

1. Improving verbal communication [3, 4]:

   (i) Teach-back method – This technique primarily asks the patient to restate what has been taught in his or her own words. This ensures that precautions, instructions, decisions or key concepts have been taught and the patient educated effectively.
   (ii) Ask Me 3 Program – Encourages patients to ask three simple questions every time a problem or concept is discussed. These questions include: (1) What is my main problem?

(2) What should I do for that problem? (3) Why is that important?

(iii) SPIKES method – This technique is helpful when communicating or discussing a difficult topic to patients and families.

(i) Setting – Provide the appropriate location for the discussion and include those that are necessary and important in the discussion.

(ii) Perception – Ensure that an accurate and appropriate picture has been painted for the patient.

(iii) Invitation – Determine the amount of information the family and patient would like to know.

(iv) Knowledge – Impart information in smaller sections and provide a setup for any bad news or information that may be discussed.

(v) Empathy – Respond to the emotional context with an appropriate, empathic response.

(vi) Strategy and summarizing – It is very important to tie together all the information and lend the patient the opportunity for questions and concerns.

(c) Team monitoring and conflict resolution [3, 4]:

(i) Situational awareness – actively scanning/assessing to gain information and understanding or awareness to support functioning of the team:

1. Cross-monitoring – Individual members monitoring others in order to reduce/avoid errors and possibly reduce workload.
2. IMSAFE tool – Structured tool; assessing status of other members once a concern arises: illness, medication, stress, alcohol /drugs, fatigue, eating, and elimination.

3. Situation monitoring is necessary to improve situational awareness. Individuals must actively scan the environment and actively listen to others, collect information, and observe other team members (cross-monitoring).
4. Multidisciplinary rounds – A group-based interactive meeting where patient care is discussed, along with any issues related to that patient's care. Although organization varies, important topics include:

   (i) Summarizing clinical data
   (ii) Identifying patient and family concerns
   (iii) Creating goals and relating progress of goals
   (iv) Highlighting current or future interventions
   (v) Analyzing and revising plan as needed
   (vi) Communicating referrals or future needs
   (vii) Reviewing discharge information
   (viii) Reviewing roles and responsibilities

5. Red rules – Red rules are a set of nonnegotiable rules communicated to team members and, in urgent situations, should almost always be followed. They must be followed by all, be enforced consistently, and be agreed upon by all group members. An example of a red rule includes always performing a time-out before any procedure is carried out.

(ii) Conflict management/team facilitation/team support [1, 2, 4]:

1. The five common methods of addressing conflict include:

   (i) Avoiding
   (ii) Accommodating
   (iii) Collaborating
   (iv) Compromising
   (v) Competing

2. Sources of conflict:
   (i) Role ambiguity/overlap in roles
   (ii) Disagreements in goals or poor clarification
   (iii) Scarcity of resources
   (iv) Difference in perceived status
   (v) Task interdependence
   (vi) Personal preferences
3. Ways to address disruptive behavior:
   (i) Acknowledge the problem.
   (ii) Establish a zero-tolerance policy.
   (iii) Maintain a code of conduct.
   (iv) Create a means to monitor and enforce certain behavior.
   (v) Educate staff on the consequences of disruptive behavior.
   (vi) Develop appropriate responses to a particular behavior.

(iii) Support tools [3, 4]:

1. Team assistance – This involves actively seeking or offering support to avoid failure, especially during periods of overload.
2. Two-challenge rule (also known as the two-attempt rule) – A communication process that seeks to ensure patient safety by empowering an individual to voice any concern that has not been addressed satisfactorily up the chain of command until a consensus has been achieved. This method directs team members to voice their concerns at least twice to ensure its acknowledgment, and recipient must return acknowledgment; failure must lead to a stronger course of action/chain of command. An assertive communication style in combination with the use of CUS words (see below) can make for more effective use of the two-challenge rule.

3. Collaboration – This includes developing solutions that meet common goals and including the patient in on decisions when appropriate.
4. CUS – Using key words to raise awareness → I am concerned, I am uncomfortable, this is a safety issue.
5. DESC – A structured, assertive communication approach for managing and resolving interpersonal conflict. DESC includes describing the situation, expressing concerns about the action, and suggesting alternatives and consequences stated – often used between team members who may be threatening each other's ability to perform. Key points to utilizing this tool effectively include framing problems in one's own experience, keeping the discussion timely, using "I" statements to minimize defensiveness, avoiding blaming statements, and focusing on what is right and not who is right.

If you have any questions about the information covered in this chapter or other medical safety and quality improvement-related topics, please contact us at http://www.medicalqualityandsafetyforum.com. The website will also provide a forum where you can ask specific questions about your safety and medical quality improvement projects or mentor upcoming medical quality leaders.

References

1. Gordon Mosser, James W. Begun. *Understanding teamwork in healthcare*. (McGraw-Hill Professional First Edition, August 2013)
2. Shirley D. *Project management for healthcare*. (Taylor and Francis Group, Boca Raton, Florida, 2011)
3. Alan H. Rosenstein, Michelle O'Daniel, Professional Communication and Team Collaboration. *Patient safety and*

quality: An Evidence-Based Handbook for Nurses. (Rockville, Maryland, Agency for Healthcare Research and Quality (US), April 2008)

4. Joint Commission on Accreditation of Healthcare Organizations. *The joint commission guide to improving staff communication*. Oakbrook Terrace, IL: Joint Commission Resources; 2005.
5. Chassin MR, Loeb JM. High-reliability Health Care: getting there from here. *Milbank* Q. 2013;91(3):459–90.

Project Management: Basics

Solomon Rojhani

Tools
Global 8D, Brainstorming, Brainwriting, Affinity diagram, Relationship map, Pareto chart, Fishbone diagram, Ishikawa diagram, Check sheet, Control chart, Histogram, Flowchart, Scatter diagram, Nominal group technique, Delphi, Cost-benefit analysis, Multivoting, Force-field diagram, Force-field analysis, Interrelationship diagram, Gantt chart, Tree diagram

There are many tools available to aid in creating, organizing, and analyzing quality improvement projects. This section demonstrates the value of several fundamental tools and incorporates the running model of the lemonade stand to aid in visualization.

S. Rojhani (✉)
Department of Physical Medicine and Rehabilitation, The Johns Hopkins University School of Medicine,
600 North Wolfe Street Phipps 160, Baltimore, MD 21287, USA
e-mail: srojhan1@jhmi.edu

L. Atanelov (ed.), *Resident's Handbook of Medical Quality and Safety*, DOI 10.1007/978-3-319-24190-6_26

Project Management Skills and Visual Tools

(a) Initiation/start – The beginning is often prompted by a goal or problem. Development of the project is discussed elsewhere in this handbook although the stages of any project often include initiating, planning, executing, monitoring and controlling, and closing [1]. The degrees of initiation vary greatly and are dependent on the needs of the team/leaders and the nature of the problem:

   (i) "Magic formula" – In this scenario, the problem is defined and a decision is then made regarding how to solve the problem.

      1. The difficulties with this method are obvious as the task is oversimplified and not intuitively informative.
      2. The "magic formula" is simple and can be applied universally and quite rapidly as exemplified below:

         (i) Problem: Individuals arriving after closing would like to be served
         (ii) Solution: an on-the-spot decision is made to stop serving 5 min after closing time and without further analysis or data collection on the problem

   (ii) "More traditional" – Here, the problem is defined, data is collected, solutions are developed, and the most appropriate solution is chosen. The winning solution is being subsequently implemented.
   (iii) "More complex" – These techniques involve greater detail. An example in this case might look like the "Eight Disciplines Problem Solving" or "Global 8D" [2]:

      1. A general outline follows the "plan-do-check-act" cycle, which has been used for years in the product development and improvement process:

(i) D0 – Initial planning stage
(ii) D1 – Establishment of a team
(iii) D2 – Problem description and goal identification
(iv) D3 – Problem containment stage to isolate the problem
(v) D4 – Identification of the root cause
(vi) D5 – Search for corrections to the problem
(vii) D6 – Implement corrective actions analysis
(viii) D7 – Prevent recurrence of the problem
(ix) D8 – Team reward for a job well done

(b) Initial planning and simple visualization:

(i) Brainstorming [3, 4]:

1. This is a commonly used forum for idea generation.
2. Several people in a group are able to build up on each other's ideas in order to maximize creativity.
3. Participants freely share ideas onto a medium. Commonly used techniques to achieve success include maintaining a criticism-free zone, having a predefined goal/problem, allowing individuals and the group time to complete idea generation period, and utilizing small groups. Brainstorming is often easy to organize and conduct (Fig. 1).

(ii)Brainwriting 6-3-5 [5, 6]:

1. This is a technique of idea generation that highlights quantity of topics generated.
2. It is an offshoot of brainstorming that aims to generate 108 different ideas within 30 min, focusing on quantity more so than quality.
3. Six participants in the group plus a moderator: each participant develops three ideas every 5 min; ideas are then written down and passed to the next individual – participants effectively inspired by each other's ideas and encouraged to constantly

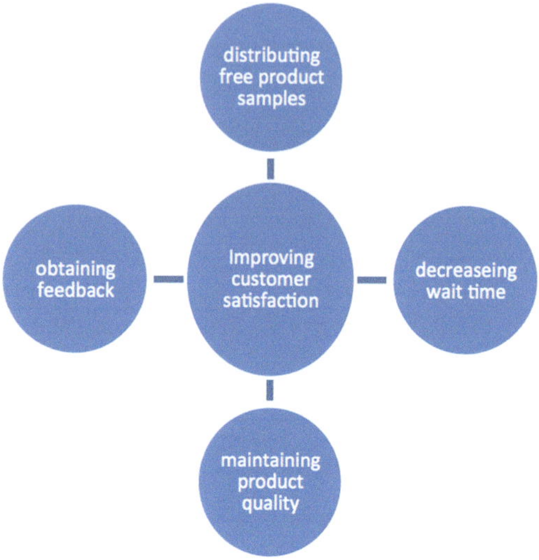
distributing free product samples
obtaining feedback
Improving customer satisfaction
decreaseing wait time
maintaining product quality

Fig. 1 Referring back to our improving customer satisfaction at our fictional lemonade stand example, ideas have been placed around a central topic in a simple, easy-to-read configuration

reinterpret and innovate off said ideas – complete 6 rounds, totaling 30 min, 108 ideas.

(iii) Affinity diagram [2, 5]:

1. A visual map comprised of the planned output of what is usually a team-based brainstorming session. Often, there is a premeditated problem/question/goal.
2. This device collectively brings together multiple often disorganized plans to create categorical structure of organized thoughts regarding a particular problem.
3. The plan of action is usually as follows: agreement on the problem and development of a question, recording of ideas onto medium, subsequent organization of thoughts and ideas, creation of headers and effectively categorizing ideas under

each header, drawing the affinity map and encapsulating each grouping, and discussion of recorded ideas/groups (Fig. 2).

(iv) Relationship diagram [2, 5]:

1. A visual tool used to evaluate cause and effect in systems, in addition to highlighting the complexity of intersystem relationships.
2. Allows for visualization of relationships between ideas in an affinity map or product of brainstorming.
3. Affinity map ideas are drawn in a circular fashion around the problem. Group members then go through interrelationships between ideas and problems or questions being asked, with cause and effect relationships being one of the more common relationships displayed (Fig. 3).

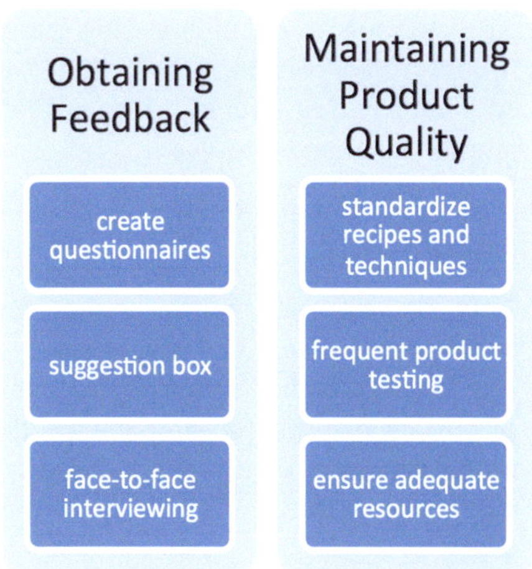

Fig. 2 A visual representation of a simple affinity diagram related to improving specific parameters regarding lemonade stand operations. The visual representation includes headers above in larger font with details pertaining to each header listed below

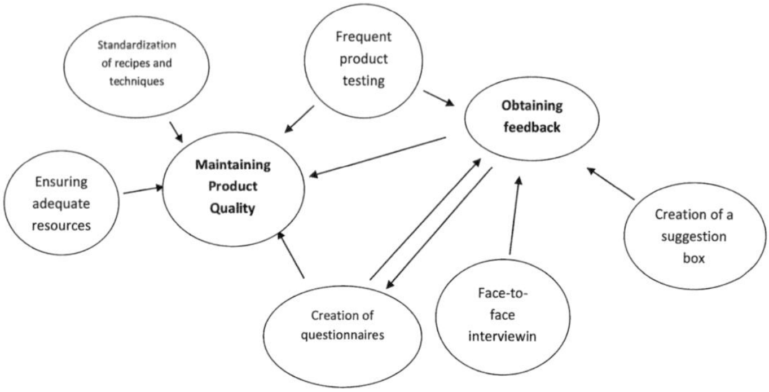

Fig. 3 Mapping a relationship diagram may be used to display cause and effect or simply display idea interrelationships

(c)Seven basic tools of quality – Originally introduced to improve quality in the engineering community, the tools include fishbone diagram, check sheet, control chart, histogram, Pareto chart, scatter diagram, and flowchart. Developed with relative simplicity in mind, these include several graphical tools to aid in assessing issues related to planning, quality control, and quality improvement. This list is by no means exhaustive and does not address more advanced statistical analytic tools [7]:

(i) Fishbone diagram/Ishikawa diagram/cause and effect diagram [2, 7, 8]:

1. This diagram aids in the evaluation of causes related to an effect.
2. The key idea is that each category can be a source of variation ultimately influencing the problem/goal. The causes/categories are usually discovered via brainstorming or other previously defined tools.
3. A problem/question/goal is defined and categories that introduce variation in different settings. The settings and their corresponding variations may include the "6 Ms" in manufacturing (machine, method, material, man power, measurement, and mother nature), or the "7 Ps" in marketing (prod-

uct, price, place, promotion, people, positioning, and packaging), and the "5 Ss" in the service industry (surroundings, suppliers, system, skills, and safety). We highlight three of the "5 Ss" in the fishbone diagram below to demonstrate its effectiveness (Fig. 4).

(ii)Check sheet [2, 7]:

1. Check sheets are commonly used tools to record data for analysis. They also provide historical records and tabulated data through various organizational methods.
2. Information may be tabular or graphical and usually presented in a simple, user-friendly fashion with clear labeling.
3. A check sheet is often used when data can be readily observed and tabulated. Data is often

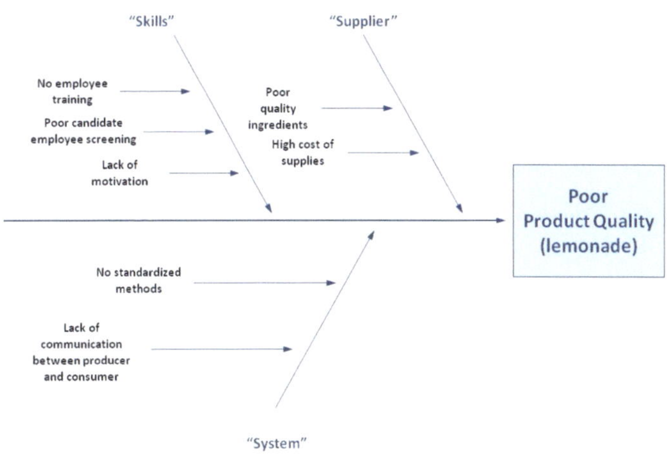

Fig. 4 Here displayed are several of the "5 Ss" to demonstrate the value of a fishbone diagram in presenting information with cause and effect relationships in mind. The causes in this case ultimately lead to poor product quality

reported in frequency of events/problems/incidences and often arises from a process involving production of a part or element.

4. A check sheet can be created as part of the evaluation of an event or problem. A decision on the length of data collection is then decided upon. The intake form should be set up so that the data is recorded simply (i.e., by Xs, Os, or check marks). Then, labels should be set up and the check sheet tested for a certain time period to measure appropriateness. Record data as the problems or events occur (Fig. 5).

(iii)Control chart [7]:

1. Helps analyze processes with variability over time and compares these data points to upper, lower and average controlled values.
2. Differentiates common from uncommon causes of variation and assesses the effectiveness of change while conveying process performance and monitoring the variation over time.
3. Control charts are able to help identify issues as they affect processes. The ranges of values are often highlighted, as well as the stability and patterns associated with a particular process.

Lemonade Purchases					
	Day				
Time	Monday	Tuesday	Wednesday	Thursday	Friday
9AM – 12PM	II	I	III	II	II
12PM – 3PM	III	IIII	II	I	IIII
3PM – 6PM	I	III	I	III	IIII

FIG. 5 A check sheet created in order to figure out the peak times of lemonade purchasing done by consumers

4. The basic process begins with choosing the appropriate control chart and determining the time period and data to be studied. Comparisons are made between data points and time while displaying upper control, lower control, and average lines. Continuously recalculate the "out-of-control" data and investigate causes (Fig. 6).

(iv)Histogram [1, 2, 7]:

1. This tool represents a bar graph of arranged data.
2. Histograms help depict a snapshot of the data pertaining to a particular process, summarizes large data sets by visualizing data distribution, compares measurements/specs, communicates information, and may assist in the decision-making process.
3. A short description of the process includes first collecting data points from a particular process. The next step often includes counting data points and using a tally process in order to create bins (as demonstrated below). Bins contain the data range, made appropriate to fit the data set. This is often complemented by determining intervals (width/starting points), counting the frequency of values within each bin, and finally plotting the data (Fig. 7).

(v)Pareto chart – originally based on the "80/20 rule of Pareto" (80 % of wealth held by 20 % of people) [2, 7]:

1. This is a bar chart arranged in descending height from left to right with relatively more important data on the left. Classically, the bars are used to represent frequency and money.
2. Helps identify most significant issues and breaks larger problems into smaller sections, at the same time designating where efforts should be focused. The ultimate result is better use of limited resources.

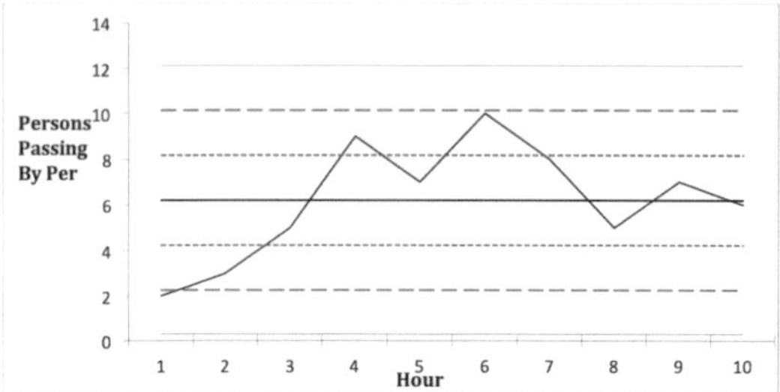

Number of Customers Passing By Per Hour on 1/1/14	
Time	Number of Individuals
8AM - 9AM	2
9AM - 10AM	3
10AM - 11AM	5
11AM - 12PM	9
12PM - 1PM	7
1PM - 2PM	10
2PM - 3PM	8
3PM - 4PM	5
4PM - 5PM	7
5PM - 6PM	6

FIG. 6 The basic visual presentation of a control chart based on tabulated data is achieved. This is an oversimplified version intended to demonstrate the value of the visual tool in graphically displaying variability of data. The average has been calculated based on tabulated data. See caption for further information. Charted data appears based on Table 26.2 on the right side of the page. The *black line* represents the average. Gradually enlarging dotted-to-solid lines represent standard deviations from the norm, beginning with one SD represented by fine dots to three SD represented by the *solid line*

3. A model for a Pareto chart begins with a categorized data, usually including but not limited to frequency, quantity, cost, and/or time. Typical time periods may include a work length, full day or week/month. Data is then recorded and organized into a graph with the maximum value or

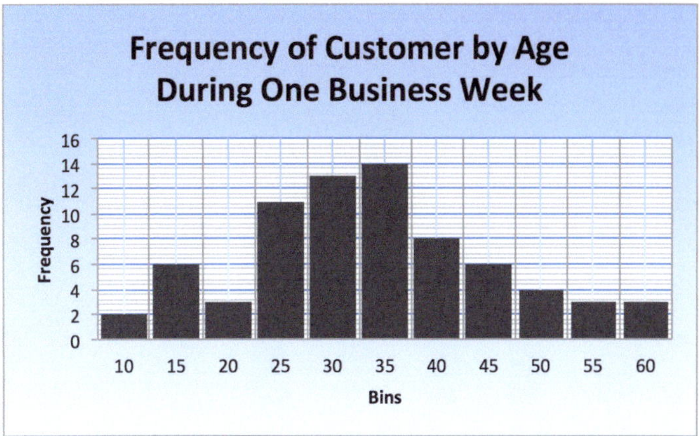

FIG. 7 This histogram represents the customer frequency based on age. Seventy-five data points have been plotted with bins organized in 5-year intervals. Our histogram may reveal a pattern of age distribution among customers to the lemonade stand and ultimately affect further business models

tallest value to the left and subsequent values arranged to the right and so on. Each category percentage should then be calculated and cumulative sums are plotted and the data points are connected (Fig. 8).

(vi)Scatter diagram [7]:

1. A scatter diagram is often utilized to study relationships between two different variables.
2. Interrelationships between variables are visualized by incorporating data from different sets on a grid in order to identify changes in the relationships of those variables over time.
3. Creation of a scatter diagram begins with a summary of tabular data. The data points are then plotted with the x-axis usually identified as the cause and the y-axis related to the effect. Data points are then plotted and trend lines may be

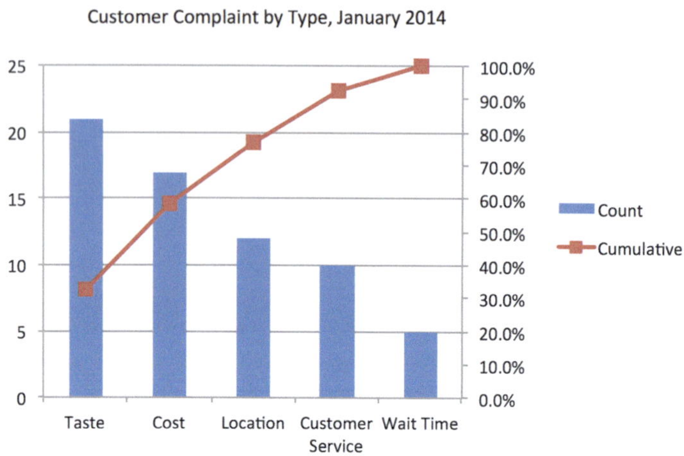

Fig. 8 The most important customer complaints, arranged in the order of significance, are highlighted. Additionally shown is a line graph representing the cumulative percentage associated with each subsequent complaint

added to better visualize the direction and strength of the correlation (Fig. 9).

(vii) Flowchart/run chart/stratification chart [7]:

1. Diagrams the nature/progression of steps in a process.
2. Flowcharts are reliable tools for training, promoting process, understanding, and identifying the problems and areas needing improvement.
3. The first step in creating a flowchart is defining the process, in addition to creating a beginning and end point. Often, it may be beneficial to write ideas down in a brainstorming session prior to creating the flowchart. To complete the chart, sequence the ideas and draw in arrows to present the direction of ideas (Fig. 10).

(d) Deciding and executing:

(i) Nominal group technique [4, 7]:

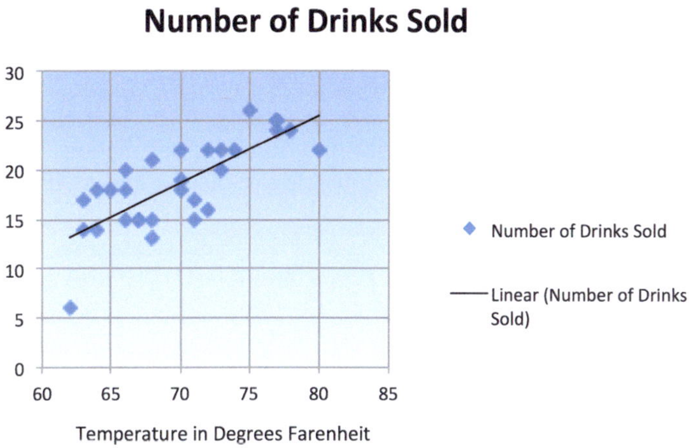

FIG. 9 A scatter diagram relating information regarding the ambient temperature and the number of drinks sold during the day. A clear trend is observed on hotter days, when desire and demand for a beverage may increase

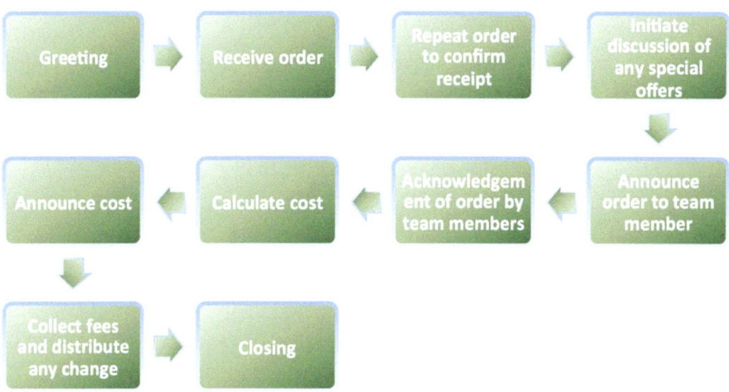

FIG. 10 A flowchart that may be shown to newly hired employees in order to provide a visual example of the order intake process, beginning from customer presentation to the stand. The chart may highlight areas of the interaction which need to be addressed prior to an adequate order intake

1. Nominal group technique (NGT) is a common method used for idea generation or decision-making.
2. NGT entails persons working in the presence of one another with only minimal interaction. This may be more appropriate than other methods when some individuals are significantly more vocal than others or when individuals prefer to work in silence. Being based on written responses, NGT may be more appropriate in the discussion of controversial topics by avoiding or lessening the dominance of individual group members. NGT is structured and easy to organize, and peer influence is still a factor in group discussion stage, although less than with other methods.
3. Decision-making via NGT begins with clarification of the statement or question, followed by silent deliberation and independent idea generation for a fixed time period. Members may then go through ideas one individual at a time while a moderator records ideas. Discussion is not encouraged at this point in time and any participant may pass his or her turn to add additional ideas. Upon completion of answer generation, a discussion is held to review each response. Final lists may be created by a technique such as multivoting to narrow down choices.

(ii) Delphi [4, 7]:

1. The Delphi technique is a means of information gathering or decision-making among a group. Responses or answers to questions and problems are collected over several rounds of questionnaires and does so anonymously. Originally developed as a means for an expert panel to face problematic issues. An in-person group meeting is not always required.

2. The workings of the Delphi technique usually include multiple rounds of question asking, with responses subsequently gathered and data recorded. Responses are read aloud so as to attempt to influence thought processes of present individuals. These results are redistributed; often revised and new sets of data are created and recorded. Groups may prioritize each answer or comment, and often an agreement may be reached by consensus, voting, or averaging. The concept here essentially remains that group decisions are commonly more significant than individual decisions.

(iii) Cost-benefit analysis (CBA) [2, 9]:

1. Includes any number of projects that compare the potential costs and benefits of a given decision or plan. CBA aims to understand the soundness of a given action in addition to acting as a basis of comparison between competing ideas or projects.
2. Consider the cost-benefit matrix below. It can help identify "low-hanging fruit." See Table 1.

(iv)Multivoting [7]:

1. This is a tool used to narrow down large lists into smaller, more manageable groups. Multivoting is often used after brainstorming to cut down large lists and when group judgment is necessary.
2. Multivoting begins with exposing previously organized options to group members and designation

Table 1 This matrix is an over-simplified representation of a cost-benifit comparison. The table visually highlights desired options or outcomes

	Low cost	**High cost**
High benefit	**Best option**	
Low benefit		

of final list size. Options are usually numbered and each member given a certain quota of choices to vote for. Essentially, the longer the list, the more votes allowed. Each member then selects and ranks the most important choices based on the number of choices allowed. The group subsequently tallies votes and records final choices with discussion then ensuing.

(v) Force-field diagram/force-field analysis [1, 7]:

1. The concept of a force-field diagram is rooted in decision-making based on comparing the forces behind each choice. Forces behind each choice can be weighted based on the importance of factors inherent to each of the forces. This is often shown by having forces on either side of the diagram, with more impactful forces being drawn in larger and broader (arrows) than less impactful forces.
2. The factors or forces must be weighted carefully and skillfully; decisions are often subjective and significant participant influence is needed. Expert judgment is often needed to give strength to subjective matter (Fig. 11).

(vi) Interrelationship diagram/relations diagram – inherently similar to a relationship map [1, 2, 7]:

1. Incorporates cause and effect relationship analysis via linking different aspects of situations.
2. This diagram is primarily used when a complex issue is being analyzed for causes and a complex solution is required, more completely exploring the relations of an idea to help make a more educated decision.
3. Begin by writing the main objective at the top of the medium and brainstorm ideas. Ideas may be incorporated from other sources such as affinity map/fishbone diagram. Relationship of each idea

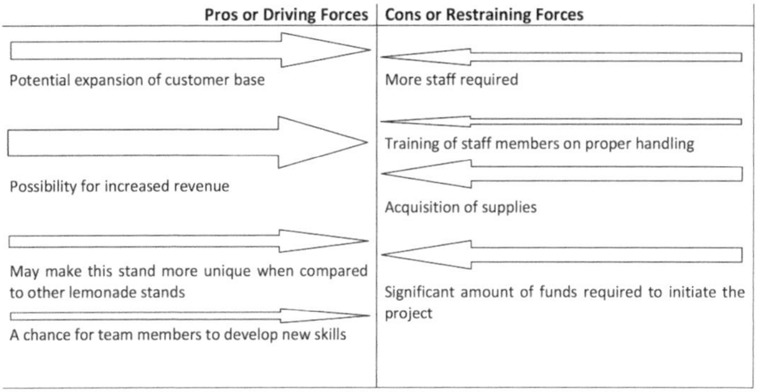

FIG. 11 In this example, the pros and cons of incorporating food items for purchase at the lemonade stand are weighed out to demonstrate the value of a force-field analysis. More significant ideas are related to *broader arrows*

to other ideas is then discussed and arranged on the medium accordingly. Arrows are then drawn to determine cause and effect relationship between ideas. The next step includes counting arrows to determine which ideas are critical. Outgoing arrows usually relate cause while incoming arrows relate effect.

(e) Implementing:

(i) Activity network diagram (also known as an Arrow Diagram and similar to the Critical Path Method) [2, 7]:

1. Defines order of tasks, scheduling, and relationship to resources.
2. This setup is useful when the steps, sequences, and duration of the project or process are known. Usually project schedule is quite critical and timing is everything.
3. Developing the diagram begins with listing of necessary tasks and orienting sequences (which

tasks should be done before? during? immediately after?). Tasks are then diagramed (timing is usually carried out from left to right). Using circles to highlight events, "dummy" events may also be added to represent potential distractions from the main or critical path (Fig. 12).

(ii)Gantt chart [7]:

1. A Gantt chart graphically displays a project timeline and the major activities that make up the timeline.
2. Normally organized by time, duration, and completion status. Useful for scheduling or monitoring tasks and conveying status or plans. The sequence and duration must be known. The order of events may or may not be dependent on completion of previous tasks.
3. The first step includes identifying tasks and the associated milestones and duration of each task. The x-axis often represents time, while the y-axis represents tasks. Status bars are then created and filled in horizontally according to task completion or projected completion dates (Fig. 13).

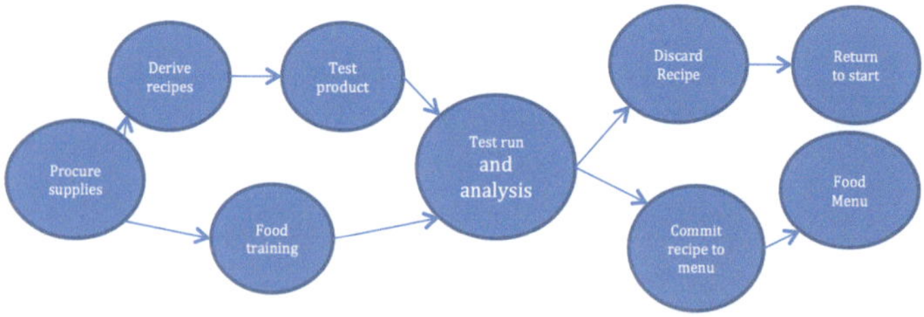

FIG. 12 An oversimplified version of an activity network diagram. Tasks are emphasized within *circles* and *arrows* to represent workflow. Additionally, timing of each task may be filled in alongside arrows to indicate task duration. Longer paths often require more time to complete tasks. Our example utilizes the basic path to adding food items to the menu

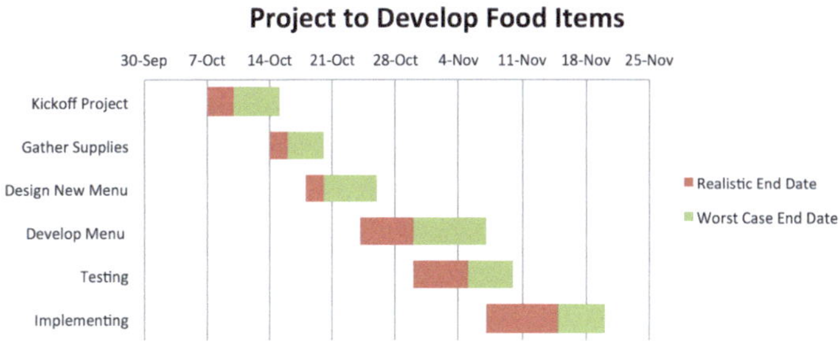

Fig. 13 The Gantt chart serves to demonstrate the timeline of events in a project to develop food items at our stand. Realistic task end dates are highlighted in *red*, while the worst case end dates of each task can be seen in *green*

(iii) Tree diagram [7]:

1. A visual tool to help assessments move from general to a more specific thinking. May be used to evaluate implementation of ideas and consequences.
2. By breaking down broad categories into increasingly detailed ideas, a tree diagram forms a branching pattern of construction to aid in visualization, develops actions to deliver a plan, and may also be used for root-cause analysis, process analysis, evaluating, and communication development. The tree diagram is truly versatile.
3. Creation of a tree diagram begins under guidance of a general statement, problem, or goal. Specific tasks are required to accomplish this idea. Those tasks or actions may be decided upon via techniques such as brainstorming, affinity diagrams, relationship diagram, or other idea-generating methods. Further levels of detail will subsequently be achieved and each idea can be evaluated and reevaluated in order to be deemed necessary and efficient (Fig. 14).

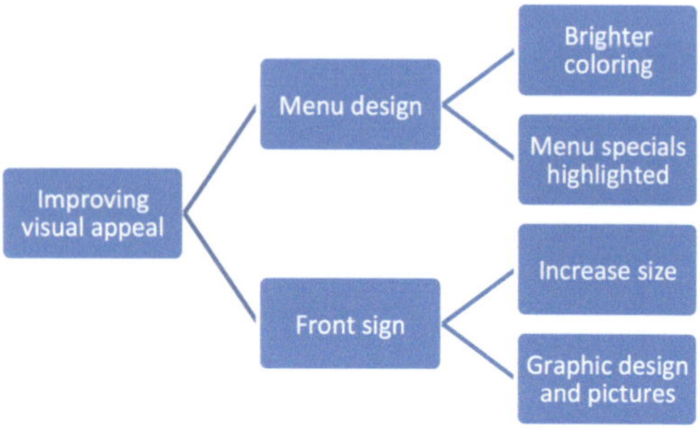

Fig. 14 This tree diagram is based on the goal of improving visual appeal at the lemonade stand. The result is the generation of several ideas to be implemented that ultimately accomplish this goal

If you have any questions about the information covered in this chapter or other medical safety and quality improvement-related topics, please contact us at http://www.medicalqualityandsafetyforum.com. The website will also provide a forum where you can ask specific questions about your safety and medical quality improvement projects or mentor upcoming medical quality leaders.

References

1. Project Management Institute. Project management body of knowledge (PMBOK guide). Newtown Township: Project Management Institute; 2013.
2. Shirley D. Project management for healthcare. Boca Raton: Taylor and Francis Group; 2011.
3. Tomas S. Creative problem-solving: an approach to generating ideas. Hosp Mater Manage Q. 1999;20(4):33–45.
4. McMurray A. Three decision-making aids: brainstorming, nominal group, and Delphi technique. J Nurs Staff Dev. 1994;10(2):62–5.
5. Lepley C. Problem-solving tools for analyzing system problems: the affinity map and the relationship diagram. J Nurs Adm. 1998;28(12):44–50.

6. Linsey JS, Becker B. Effectiveness of brainwriting techniques: comparing nominal groups to real teams. In: Taura T, Nagai Y, editors. Design creativity 2010. London: Springer; 2011. 166 p.
7. Tague N. The quality toolbox. 2nd ed. Milwaukee: ASQ Quality Press; 2004.
8. Ishikawa K, Loftus JH, editors. Introduction to quality control. Tokyo: 3A Corporation; 1990.
9. Jeremy J, Duncan H. Qualitative research: consensus methods for medical and health services research. BMJ. 1995;311:376.

Team Management in Healthcare: Basics

Solomon Rojhani

Tools
Team building, Tuckman's stages of group development, Belbin's team roles, TeamSTEPPS

Teamwork in Healthcare

(i) Building an effective team:

1. A project manager has a "homework" prior to building a team [1]. He must be able to:

    (i) Define mission, goals, and objectives related to the project.
    (ii) Align the team with the goals in mind.
    (iii) Prepare to nurture a motivational environment.
    (iv) Communicate effectively to team members.
    (v) Define roles and responsibilities/assignments.

S. Rojhani (✉)
Department of Physical Medicine and Rehabilitation, The Johns Hopkins University School of Medicine,
600 North Wolfe Street Phipps 160, Baltimore, MD 21287, USA
e-mail: srojhan1@jhmi.edu

L. Atanelov (ed.), *Resident's Handbook of Medical Quality and Safety*, DOI 10.1007/978-3-319-24190-6_27

(vi) Define a conflict resolution strategy.
(vii) Create rewards.
(viii) Understand Tuckman's original stages of group development, which are the basis for growth and development and team problem solving. This model includes "forming-storming-norming-perfoming" [2].

2. Team forming/planning includes asking basic questions of a team and its members [3]. A sample battery of relevant questions may include:

   (i) What are the tasks?
   (ii) Who are the other members?
   (iii) Will I like working with these members? Will they like working with me?
   (iv) What is expected of me? What do I expect from others?
   (v) How will the team affect my daily work?
   (vi) How significant is leadership? What is the expected level of competency? What types of personalities will I encounter?

3. Storming: Initial group-forming stages are marked by clashing of personalities. A commonly used analogy that reflects this idea pertains to passengers on a lifeboat. This analogy entails the idea that on a lifeboat at sea, there may be those individuals who are "fire starters," others who are "gasoline throwers," and yet others who are constantly extinguishing these flames. Leadership is thus important to get to the norming stage of development. Additionally, leaders must manage criticism well as there may be a plethora during these stages [3, 5].
4. Norming: Here there is increased listening time and increased interpersonal understanding, and teammates begin to "get" each other. A common goal is decided upon and individuals abandon their own goals for the greater good of the team. This leads to the eventual ability to perform [3, 5].

5. Performing: At this higher level of functioning, teams are able to unite to get the job done. The team is usually able to make decisions on its own, and although criticism is expected, conflict is usually avoided or dealt with appropriately [3, 5].

(ii) Characteristics of effective teams in healthcare [3]:

1. Characteristics of effective teams in healthcare – *structure*:
   - (i) Shared goal understood by all members
   - (ii) Shared responsibility across team members for achieving the goal
   - (iii) Well-defined membership for the whole team
   - (iv) Clear leadership, acknowledged by all
   - (v) Sufficient hierarchy for quick decision-making if needed
   - (vi) Adequate authority
   - (vii) Stability of membership: the more stable the better

2. Characteristics of effective teams in healthcare – *focus*:
   - (i) Respect for the interests of patients and families, above all
   - (ii) Generation of trust in patients/families
   - (iii) Support for patients as partners in the management of their own care

3. Characteristics of effective teams in healthcare – *orientation*:
   - (i) Agreement on common values
   - (ii) Agreement on common set of processes
   - (iii) Identity of a cohesive team
   - (iv) Creation of a favorable social climate
   - (v) Mutual accountability
   - (vi) Team building/maintaining activities

4. Characteristics of effective teams in healthcare – *collaboration*:

    (i) Respect by all for all.
    (ii) Trust among the members.
    (iii) Active interdependence and reliability.
    (iv) Evidence-based medicine as a foundation.
    (v) Effective communication.
    (vi) Prevent/manage conflict.

5. Characteristics of effective teams in healthcare – *team management*:

    (i) See below.

(iii) Team roles – often initially defined by an individual's interests/competencies [3]:

1. Five occupational interests:

    (i) Realistic occupation (practical/hands-on/individual/raw material)
    (ii) Investigative (critical thinking/working with ideas)
    (iii) Artistic (forms/designs and patterns/self-expression)
    (iv) Social (communicating/teaching/providing service)
    (v) Enterprising (starting up/carrying out projects/decisions/risk taking/business)

2. In healthcare this often becomes the five professions, including medicine, nursing, pharmacy, social work, and healthcare administration.

    (i) Must have the six common goals in mind:

        (i) Safety
        (ii) Effectiveness
        (iii) Patient centeredness
        (iv) Timeliness
        (v) Efficiency
        (vi) Equity

3. Values of individual – preference regarding appropriate course of action/outcomes + occupational interest(s) = profile.
4. Belbin's team roles – include additional ways to categorize individual personalities: innovator, resource investigator, coordinator, shaper, monitor/evaluator, team worker, implementer, completer/finisher, and specialist.

(iv) Essentials regarding momentum/motivation [1, 3, 5]:

1. Mayo 1927 – group interaction, affiliation, and personal attention of management are bigger influences than salary/benefits.
2. Herzberg 1968 – motivation-hygiene theory: motivators (real stimulus) and hygiene (dissatisfiers if not present but do not directly stimulate employee productivity):

   (i) Motivators – sense of achievement, recognition by management, work itself, responsibility, advancement, and personal growth
   (ii) Hygiene – company policy, micromanagement, working conditions, and salary

3. Maslow hierarchy – by ascertaining where a team member is located on the hierarchy scale, motivation becomes more manageable, as the needs of an individual may be properly addressed. Listed below are the qualities Maslow originally described followed by a brief description of examples of needs within the hierarchy [3, 4]:

   (i) Physiological/bodily needs – basics for life (e.g., food, water, sleep, etc.)
   (ii) Safety/security – job security, retirement plan, and life insurance
   (iii) Love/belonging – affiliation, community, and relationships
   (iv) Esteem – recognition, appreciation, reputation, confidence, competence, and dignity

(v) Self-actualization – most complex: completeness, fulfillment, and creativity. See Fig. 1.

(v)Team creativity [2, 3]:

1. Denotes different qualities from individual creativity:

   (i) Individuals are inherently more creative, divergent, and explorative thinkers. Team thinking may be more critical, convergent, and marked by exploitation.

2. Team must be able to understand creativity as a goal and maintain certain ideals:

   (i) Not an easily achievable goal: ideas need to be creative yet realistic.
   (ii) Diversity should be encouraged by appointing members with a wide spectrum of perspectives/

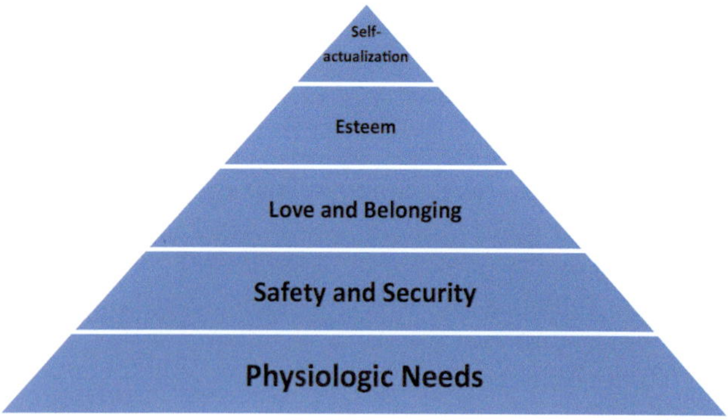

Fig. 1 Maslow plotted a hierarchy of needs whereby individuals are motivated the highest level, termed "self-actualization." The five-stage model can be divided into basic needs (e.g., physiological, safety, love, and esteem) and growth development (self-actualization). A person must satisfy more basic needs before progressing on to meet higher level growth needs. Once these needs have been reasonably fulfilled, one may be able to reach the highest level, called self-actualization

creative styles. Strive for moderate turnover and decrease socialization of new members.

(iii) Support creativity by building participation, positivity toward problem solving, being the “yes” man, reviewing, and reflecting upon ideas.

(iv) Increase the base of knowledge by studying best practices, positive deviations, brainstorming, and other methods as described.

(v) Challenge each other by publicizing high-performance standards. Prepare participants to expect that ideas may not ever be used nor implemented.

(vi) Stop working and have fun. Use humor and balance exploitation/critical thinking/convergent thinking in combination with exploration/creative thinking/divergent thinking.

(vi) Key points regarding project management and conducting meetings [3]:

1. Unity of purpose and structure. Subgroups should not operate independently of the whole or without the larger group in mind.
2. Forming a favorable social climate.
3. Creating an enjoyable work environment and enjoyment of the actual work.
4. Effective team-building skills.
5. Effective team-level operations.
6. Conducting effective business meetings and general orders of business:

   (i) Review of minutes from previous encounter
   (ii) Incoming/outgoing correspondence
   (iii) Committee reports
   (iv) Special orders
   (v) Unfinished business – new business
   (vi) Announcements/miscellaneous

7. Managing unresolved conflict
8. Timely and effective training plan

9. Systematic performance improvement
10. Motivation and momentum
11. Sponsorship of the team
12. General support from the larger organization

(vii) Leadership:

1. Good leadership must be able to create conditions that enable team to function, build the teams capacity to do work, and coach the team to optimize performance.
2. Great man/woman theory (exceptionally influential individual) vs. trait theory (patterns of personal characteristics) vs. event theory (greatness arises amidst chaos or crisis).
3. Many comparisons can be made between a coach and a leader, and often they share the ability to radiate passion, strive for the success of the team, be a visionary, and adapt to different situations.
4. It pays to be a great enabler and developer:

    (i) Enabler – as an enabler, the individual must establish a common understanding of goals, establish shared responsibility and mutual accountability, assure sufficient team authority, establish interdependency of members, create a defined membership, maintain unification, and relate leadership to larger organization or sponsor.

    (ii) Developer – responsible for recruitment, orientation, and team formation, establish team values, assure common understanding, maintain hierarchy, foster team identity, keep favorable social climate and psychological safety, and assure effective team-level operations.

(viii) The role of TeamSTEPPS (Team Strategies to Enhance Performance and Patient Safety) [6]:

1. Developed by AHRQ (Agency of Healthcare Reform and Quality) with the goal to improve safety,

this tool encompasses five major principles including team structure, leadership, situation monitoring, mutual support, and communication. Ideas will be further elaborated in the communication chapter.

If you have any questions about the information covered in this chapter or other medical safety and quality improvement-related topics, please contact us at http://www.medicalqualityandsafetyforum.com. The website will also provide a forum where you can ask specific questions about your safety and medical quality improvement projects or mentor upcoming medical quality leaders.

References

1. Shirley D. Project management for healthcare. Boca Raton: Taylor and Francis Group Florida; 2011.
2. Tuckman B. Developmental sequence in small groups. Psychol Bull. 1965; 63(6): 384–99.
3. Mosser G, Begun JW. Understanding teamwork in health care. 1st ed. New York: McGraw-Hill Professional; 2013.
4. Project Management Institute. Project management body of knowledge (PMBOK guide). 5th ed. Newton Square: Project Management Institute; 2013.
5. Tomas S. Creative problem-solving: an approach to generating ideas. Hosp Mater Manage Q. 1999;20(4):33–45.
6. Joint Commission on Accreditation of Healthcare Organizations. The joint commission guide to improving staff communication. Oakbrook Terrace: Joint Commission Resources; 2005.

Quality Improvement Tools: A Potpourri

Charles A. Odonkor

Tools
DMAIC, fishbone diagram, PDCA, and PDSA

Introduction

What Is Improvement?

Central to the concept of improvement is the idea of change. Improvement infers a future reference state in relation to an existing state of affairs, where one expects things to have changed for the better. As previously described elsewhere, "without change, there can be no improvement." However, not all change leads to improvement. Change that results in improvement can be considered positive. Achieving positive

C.A. Odonkor (✉)
Department of Physical Medicine and Rehabilitation,
Johns Hopkins Hospital, 600 North Wolfe Street, Phipps 160,
Baltimore, MD 21287, USA
e-mail: codonko2@jhmi.edu

L. Atanelov (ed.), *Resident's Handbook of Medical Quality and Safety*, DOI 10.1007/978-3-319-24190-6_28

change requires goal setting, critical observation of the status quo and understanding what needs to change and why change needs to happen, having a mechanism to measure the intended change, test-driving the change, knowing how to implement the change, and understanding how to make the change sustainable. According to Parry et al., improvement is grounded in learning cycles [1]. These generally encompass three phases: (1) an innovation phase, (2) a testing phase, and (3) a scale-up and spread phase [2]. Accompanying each phase is a degree of belief in the intervention, with an upward gradient from low to high by the scale-up and spread phase. Thus, interventions and choice of improvement methods are guided by one's degree of belief in the effectiveness of the proposed intervention. Through systematic testing and iterative learning cycles, one becomes adept at tailoring interventions to the appropriate contexts. From a healthcare perspective, implementation of new intervention requires buy-in from multiple stakeholders. Without a degree of belief in proposed changes, an ethos of care, as well as an understanding of a health system and its culture, it becomes very difficult to effectively implement change in the care setting. Improvements in the health system involve a complex process of social change and cultural shift, requiring teamwork and stakeholder collaboration for success. In particular, those at the front line and point of care with firsthand knowledge of the issues in question are best suited to implement change through a series of plan-do-study-act cycles. It is important to note that all improvement projects have high and low points, and this feature is an anticipated part of the QI process. As such low points should not be considered signs of failure, but rather should be viewed as teachable moments. QI learning processes are discussed next.

PDCA Cycle

PDCA is a systematic framework to foster a continuum of change developed by Walter Shewhart and made popular by W. Edwards Deming [3]. PDCA was used in the manufacturing industry and had been adopted for healthcare needs [4].

The PDCA cycle applies to simple improvement scenarios and testing rounds of pilot projects, prior to system-wide implementation. The PDCA cycle churns continuously in consistent repetitive steps until the desired results are accomplished and maintained (Fig. 1). PDCA is sometimes referred to as the Deming cycle or the Deming Wheel [3].

- PDCA stands for Plan, Do, Check, Act.
- *Plan*: An action plan or intervention is generated. For the lemonade stand example, design ways to reduce customer wait times to less than 1 min after ordering.
- *Do*: The intervention is executed. Premix lemonade drinks in dispenser ready for customer orders to limit lemonade preparation and delivery time.

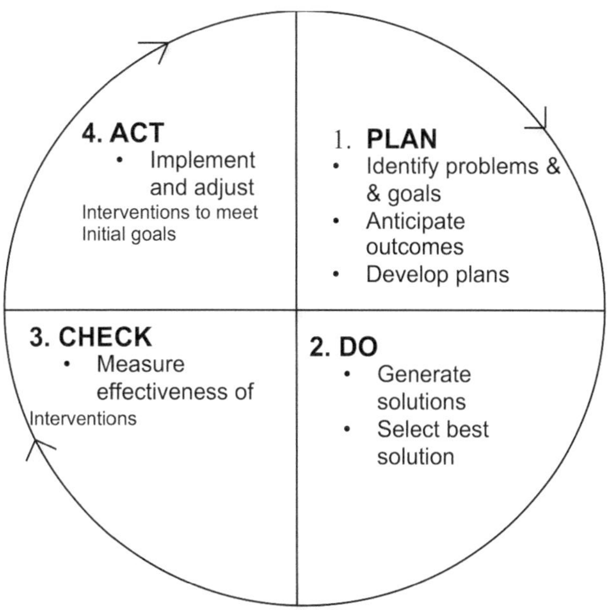

FIG. 1 PDCA cycle. This figure explains the directionality of implementing the Plan-Do-Change-Act cycle

- *Check:* The intervention is evaluated for success or failure. Does premixing reduce waiting times to less than 1 min?
- *Act:* Ideas are generated to adjust the intervention to better approximate the desired outcome. Provide customers with cups for self-dispensing of drinks.

PDSA Cycle

PDSA is very similar to the PDCA, the major difference being that PDSA is applied in more complex improvement scenarios [5].This goes beyond merely comparing the initial and end phase of one system (common to PDCA cycles) to the next step of performing more thorough reflection and contemplation of each aspect of multi-complex systems to implement new information that would help attain the desired goals for all systems. PDSA is sometimes referred to as the Shewhart cycle. PDCA cycle may be viewed as the nascent stage preceding PDSA cycle.

- PDSA stands for Plan, Do, Study, Act.
- *Plan*: An action plan or interventions are generated.
- *Do*: Interventions are executed.
- *Study:* Different levels of interventions are evaluated for success or failure.
- *Act:* Ideas are generated to adjust the interventions to better approximate the desired outcomes (Fig. 1).

DMAIC

DMAIC is an abbreviation which stands for Define, Measure, Analyze, Improve, Control and refers to a data-driven quality improvement framework often used with Six Sigma methodology developed to minimize variability in processes. The Six Sigma tool was originally developed by Motorola in the 1980s to reduce product variation [5, 6]. DMAIC provides a basic structure for Six Sigma implementation by providing a systematic approach to quality improvement projects. DMAIC is not exclusive to Six Sigma and can be used as the framework for other improvement applications. For example, DMAIC has been adapted to healthcare to guide healthcare improvement and patient safety initiatives [7]. As an illustration of DMAIC, consider the following:

- *Define the problem at hand.* For the lemonade stand example, two problems could be defined: (1) customers are spending too much time waiting in-line to order and (2) there is too much variability in lemonade sweetness per serving. Say on average, your ideal customer wait time is 120 s, and currently customers spend 480 s waiting in-line (alternatively, given that there may not be an ideal wait time, a good goal would be say cutting down wait times by about 50 %), or that the standard sugar content per 8 fl oz serving (cup) of lemonade is 25 g, but there are some servings that have either less (10 g) or more (40 g) sugar, so your goal would be to eliminate this variability and to cut down wait times. The expected benefit is a standardized product with less variability in sugar content.
- *Measure current baseline.* For example, how much sugar content is in each drink per serving? Let's say you know that a standard bottle (500 ml) of lemonade contains 70 g of sugar, but you want to produce a product with 10 % less sugar content for a serving (250 ml cup). Normally the 250 ml of lemonade would have half the sugar content, 35 g = ([250/500] × 70), but you want 10 % less sugar, so this would be [35–10% (35)] = 31.5 g. To make your 240 ml lemonade with 10 % less sugar from the original stock (500 ml bottle which contains 70 g of sugar), the process would be [240 ml × 31.5g] / 70 g = 112.5 ml. So you take out 112 ml of the 500 ml lemonade drink and dilute it with 128 ml of water (240–112 = 128 ml) to obtain the new product, 240 ml lemonade, which contains only 31.5 g of sugar. This process can be applied on a larger scale to make sure all your servings (240 ml) of lemonade contain 31.5 g of sugar.

- *Analyze and identify the specific causes of the problem.* For example, you notice one source of variability in the sugar content in the lemonade drinks is the inconsistency of mixing ratios of sugar to lemon juice to water. You want to make sure that all subsequent lemonade servings have a ratio of 1:2:1. One simple fix would be to change the juicer to an automated digitized processor that squeezes the exact same amount of juice from each lemon. Use well-calibrated cups for all your measurements, and at each step, check to make sure that the correct volume of each ingredient is being measured. Take 60 ml of sugar syrup and add to 120 ml of lemon juice and 60 ml of water each time for a perfect mixing ratio of 1:2:1.
- Improve and implement the intervention to reduce the problem. Use same standard measuring tools for mixing drinks and the same mixing methods. In the above example, the automated juice and automated mixer could be simple fixes that would ensure the same mixing ratios are performed and maintained every time.
- Control to ensure that the improvement phase lasts and to ensure that deviations from goal performance are corrected without causing defects. For example, for the lemonade stand, make sure the percentage of sugar content per drink is the same by using a reliable glucometer to measure final concentration of drinks prior to serving. Each step of the process must be checked before moving to the next step. Of note, it is important to define how frequently the process of interest is monitored at this stage, e.g., use a glucometer to check every 100th lemonade produced, or have a timer go off every 40 min to remind you to NOW stop and check the glucose content of the current drink in production.
- So you check your volumes and you check your instruments to make sure they are well calibrated and measuring the correct volumes. You check your cooling conditions to make sure they are standardized and remain the same every time you prepare the lemonade. When you notice a problem, say glucometer is not accurately measuring glucose content, you either fix it or purchase a new glucometer.

In comparison to PDCA/PDSA cycles, DMAIC is part of the Six Sigma approach with a heavy focus on customer-centric measures and is particularly useful for high-frequency processes that require multiple repetitions, for example, yearly flu vaccinations, health screenings, and patient laboratory tests. Certified practitioners (often at different levels of proficiency, with the highest level being a black belt) are trained to implement all steps of DMAIC [8]. For an example of DMAIC that is relevant to a clinical scenario, see Box 1.

Box 1: DMAIC for Post-hospital Syndrome

Post-hospital syndrome is defined as an acquired transient risk experienced by patients where they are more vulnerable to illness days to weeks following a hospital stay. One contributing factor is that most patients have no form of exercise during their hospital stay and are confined to bed rest and as such are exposed to risks such as VTEs, pressure ulcers, worsened cardiopulmonary function, muscle weakness, and generalized deconditioning. One simple fix could be encouraging mobility and out of bed with ambulation as tolerated.

DMAIC addressing the above is outlined below:

Define:

- Problem: Unnecessary bed rest can be dangerous to patients.
- Goal: Unnecessary bed rest should be minimized.
- Benefit: Reduce bed rest-associated medical complications.
- Scope: Two medical-surgical nursing units.

(continued)

Box 1 (continued)
Measure:

What

- Identify causes of unnecessary bed rest and/or barriers to patient mobility.
- Measure baseline patient mobility prior to intervention.
- Measure baseline rate of medical complications and hospital length of stay.

How

- Develop a survey to assess barriers to patient mobility.
- Administer the survey to the medical care team (e.g., physicians, nurses, physical and occupational therapist) to identify baseline barriers to patient mobility.
- Develop a scale to measure patient mobility.
  - For example, a metric called highest activity level (HAL), which is now used in some hospitals, includes:
    (1) Lying in bed
    (2) In-bed activity
    (3) Sitting at the edge of bed
    (4) Transferring to a chair/commode
    (5) Static standing (1 or more minutes)
    (6) Walking ten steps or more (i.e., walking to the restroom)
    (7) Walking 25 ft or more (i.e., walking outside the room)
    (8) Walking 250 ft or more (i.e., several laps on the unit).
- Develop an electronic medical system tool to document HAL.
- Engage nursing staff to regularly document HAL.

- Educate nursing staff on the importance of tracking patient mobility.
- Measure compliance with HAL documentation requirement (three times a day per patient).
- Keep nursing staff accountable for HAL documentation.
- Provide regular feedback on HAL documentation.
- Conduct weekly meetings to discuss challenges with HAL documentation and propose solutions to these challenges.
- *You can use the PDCA** cycle framework to *plan* ways to comply with HAL documentation, *do* (execute) the discussed plans, *check* (evaluate) success of the plans, and *act* or identify corrective measures at regular meetings to improve compliance with HAL documentation.

Analyze:

What

- Analyze the survey results.
- Analyze compliance with HAL documentation.

How

- Use analysis tools such as multivariable regression to identify variables associated with barriers to patient mobility.
- Use a run chart to display compliance with HAL documentation.

(continued)

Box 1 (continued)

(Figure 2)

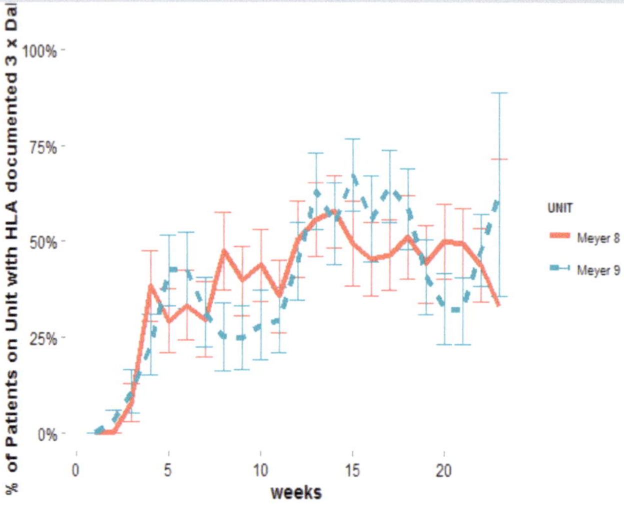

FIG. 2 Run chart. Staff adherence to documenting HAL increases with time. This figure provides an example of how a run chart can be used to track outcomes; in this case, the run chart highlights how front staff are becoming engaged with a tool by recording patients' highest activity level, and encouraging mobility and out of bed with ambulation as tolerated, to reduce post-hospital syndrome

Improve:

What

- Fluctuations in the level of compliance with HAL documentation

(continued)

Box 1 (continued)

- Road blocks to compliance with HAL documentation – understaffing and lack of incentives for staff to implement HAL

How

- Analyze barriers to HAL documentation.
- Organize regular meetings with the nursing staff to discuss challenges with HAL documentation.
- Provide incentives to staff (e.g., STAR award for staff of the month with full HAL documentation).

Control:

What

- Stakeholder support and participation.
- Resources to incentivize staff to continue implementation of HAL.
- Set unit-wide average compliance target rate.
- Set acceptable variation rate with clearly defined upper and lower limits of compliance.

How

- With stakeholder support and enough data for benefit of HAL on patient outcomes, help establish hospital policy that makes HAL documentation standard part of all patient admissions.
- Send quarterly compliance rates per unit to all units for self-monitoring of unit performance.
- Continue to encourage units to work toward a goal of establishing compliance rate (at least >80 %).
- Compare baseline (i.e., pre-intervention) patient mobility to the post-intervention level of patient mobility.

If you have any questions about the information covered in this chapter or other medical safety and quality improvement-related topics, please contact us at http://www.medicalqualityandsafetyforum.com. The website will also provide a forum where you can ask specific questions about your safety and medical quality improvement projects or mentor upcoming medical quality leaders.

References

1. Parry GJ. A brief history of quality improvement. J Oncol Pract. 2014;10(3):196–9.
2. Perla RJ, Provost LP, Parry GJ. Seven propositions of the science of improvement: exploring foundations. Qual Manag Health Care. 2013;22(3):170–86.
3. Shewhart WA (1986) Statistical method from the viewpoint of quality control. Mineola: Courier Dover Publications
4. Berwick DM. Developing and testing changes in delivery of care. Ann Intern Med. 1998;128(8):651–6.
5. Cleghorn GD, Headrick LA. The PDSA cycle at the core of learning in health professions education. Jt Comm J Qual Improv. 1996;22(3):206–12.
6. Pyzdek T, Keller PA. The six sigma handbook. New York: McGraw-Hill; 2003.
7. Antony J, Antony FJ, Kumar M, Cho BR. Six sigma in service organisations: benefits, challenges and difficulties, common myths, empirical observations and success factors. Int J Qual Reliab Manage. 2007;24(3):294–311.
8. Goldstein M (2001). Six Sigma program success factors. Six Sigma Forum Magazine, British Standards Institute

Quality Improvement (QI): Implementing QI Tools

Charles A. Odonkor

> **Tools**
> Cost-benefit matrix, Lean A3 diagram, Process flow-chart, RACI chart, Sequence of events diagram, Six Sigma, SIPOC diagram, Spaghetti diagrams, Swim lane diagram, Value stream diagram, Kanban

Introduction

As you may recall from the previous chapter, the PDCA (plan, do, control, act) is a framework for fostering a continuum of systematic change. Here we consider how to use several QI tools with the PDCA as a template.

C.A. Odonkor (✉)
Department of Physical Medicine and Rehabilitation, Johns Hopkins Hospital, 600 North Wolfe Street, Phipps 160, Baltimore, MD 21287, USA
e-mail: codonko2@jhmi.edu

L. Atanelov (ed.), *Resident's Handbook of Medical Quality and Safety*, DOI 10.1007/978-3-319-24190-6_29

Plan

1. **Identify the problem: To do this, examine processes, outcomes, systems/structures, and standards.**

   - In the arena of healthcare, stakeholders must work with frontline staff to identify the potential problem areas. According to Avedis Donabedian, the three central components of quality of care are (1) care processes, the way medical care is performed; (2) outcomes, the results of these processes; and (3) the settings/structures, where these processes take place (buildings, organizations, people) [1].
   - Addressing systems and processes is vital to quality care. Thus, the planning phase should aim at "delivery of the right intervention, at the right time, in the right place and in right manner" [2].

     (i) **Processes**:

     - A crucial part of this step involves being present at the **gemba** (Japanese for "workplace") to observe what is actually happening on the ground and to identify the potential problem areas. In the lemonade stand example, this means being present at the site of manufacturing and distribution to identify the rate-limiting steps requiring improvement.
     - Deming offers some insights into the processes when he suggests that "85 % of the reasons for failure to meet customer requirements are related to deficiencies in systems and processes… rather than the employee. The role of management is to change the process rather than badgering individuals to do better."
     - Develop a process flowchart. See example in Fig. 1 and Table 1.
     - Other alternatives of process planning tools include: SIPOC diagram (see Table 2 and Fig. 2), fishbone

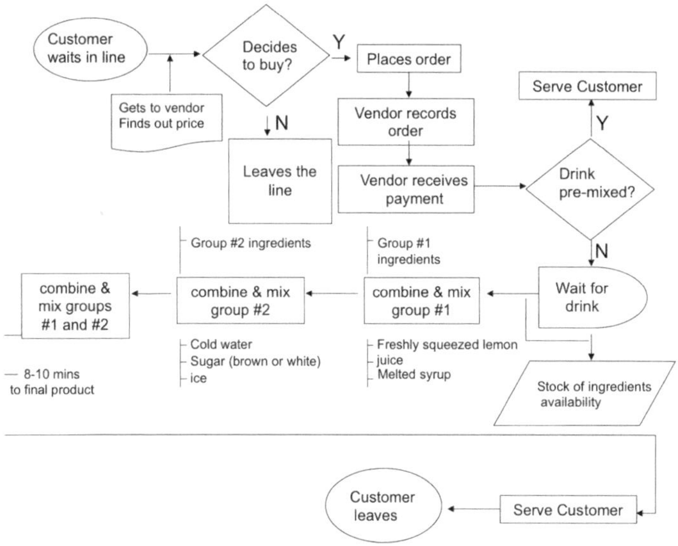

FIG. 1 Process flowchart for lemonade stand

TABLE 1 Process flowchart

What does this do? Enables visualization of the intricate steps in a process for any service or product
How does it work?
Identifies the problem areas where inefficiencies may exist. Allows conceptualization of the limits and boundaries of a process. Level of details to include in the chart may be decided upon by team members as needed to meet desired goals

diagram (also known as Ishikawa diagram or the cause-and-effect diagram) (Table 3 and Fig. 3), swim lane diagram (Table 4 and Fig. 4), value stream diagram (Table 5), and sequence of events diagram (Table 6 and Fig. 5).

TABLE 2 SIPOC diagram

What does this do? Describes the boundaries and elements of a system by defining the "suppliers," "inputs," "process," "outputs," and "customers." Clearly states the start and end points of a process. It may be helpful to create a SPICOC diagram prior to creating a fishbone diagram or process flowchart
How does it work?
Allows team members to become aligned on the scope of an improvement project, encourages delineation of the items external to the project, and keeps the group within the scope of issues under investigation

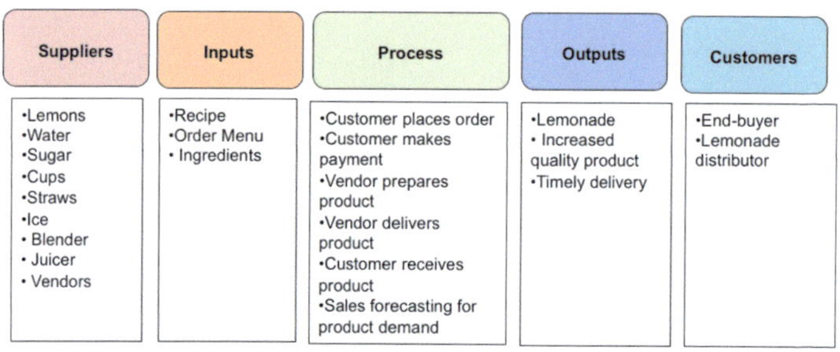

FIG. 2 SIPOC diagram. Please refer to a more conventional description of SIPOC on page 211, Editor's Note

(ii)**Outcomes:** Examine outcomes by performing root cause analysis. Here a fishbone diagram will help in delineating the relationships among various root factors underlying a problem or series of events (Fig. 3). For instance, in the lemonade stand example above, the root cause of lemonade sugar content variability could be having inadequate structure, i.e., using uncalibrated caps. Performing root cause analysis helps to clearly define the problem, identify the multifactorial constituents of the problem, mark common errors and error patterns, and develop solutions.

TABLE 3 Fishbone diagram
What does this do? Enables graphic visualization of the relationships among various root factors underlying a problem or sentinel event. One can also group different types of problems as structure (poor training, inadequate equipment, poor layout of stands, etc.) or process (unsteady provision of supplies, poor advertising technique, too much waste, too much variability, etc.) deficits contributing to deficient outcomes. Root cause definition refers to key simplest factor underlying a problem. This means breaking down an issue into key component until the problem can no longer be broken down. For example, you establish that a reason for variability in the percentage of sugar content of lemonade is lack of calibrated measuring cups to measure exact quantities of sugar
How does it work?
Identifies the range of effects and causes that generate those effects. It makes explicit the latent sources of errors via root cause analysis. These become the focal points of quality improvement projects to meet desired outcomes

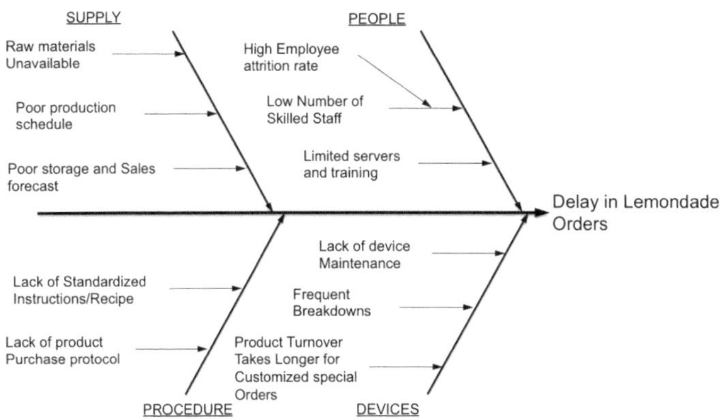

FIG. 3 Fishbone diagram for lemonade stand

TABLE 4 Swim lane diagram

What does this do? Categorizes all the steps in a process and places the identical steps in streamline paths or lanes. Allows team members to quickly identify the bottlenecks (e.g. movement of people, information and transport of materials) for process improvement
How does it work?
Places distinct tasks or steps in separate lanes and outlines the relationships among the steps. Works very similar to a flowchart, but with tasks places in specific categories

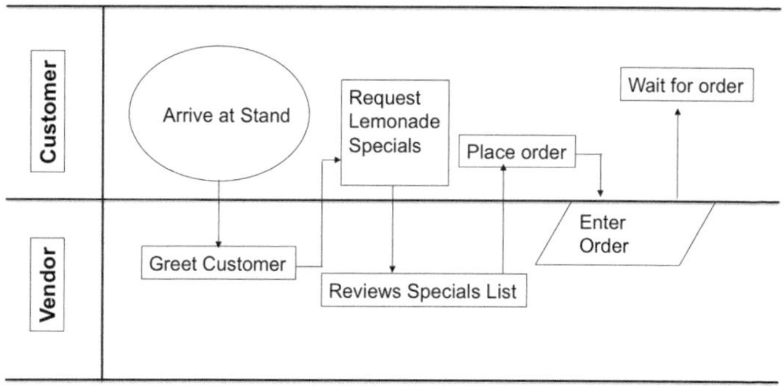

FIG. 4 Swim lane diagram

(iii) Assess the geography of where the process takes place, e.g. would it be helpful to add an extra patient care room in the emergency department or co-locate offices of people often working with each other in person. Using a Spaghetti diagram (Fig. 6) can help generate ideas.

- **Apply 5S** workplace organization theory to foster efficiency, promote a better run business, and provide a good work environment.
- 5S organization is a method borrowed from the Japanese and refers to seiri (sort), seiton (set in order), seiso (clean up), seiketsu (standardize), and shitsuke (sustain) [3].
- Recognize the interplay between organizational culture and influence of external factors. What is the

TABLE 5 Value stream diagram

What does this do? Creates an outline of the current state of a process under investigation and contrasts with a future ideal state of the process after elimination of waste and inefficiencies. This is often used by manufacturers with large-scale production plants
How does it work?
Identifies all problem areas with waste and inefficiencies and helps to find ways to eliminate these problems

TABLE 6 Sequence of events diagram

What does this do? Outlines the order in which steps in a process occur by organizing interactions between those steps in a time sequence. It highlights the temporal relationship of events and actors
How does it work?
Use parallel vertical lines (also known as lifelines) to depict different processes that occur concurrently and horizontal arrows to depict the interchange between sequenced events

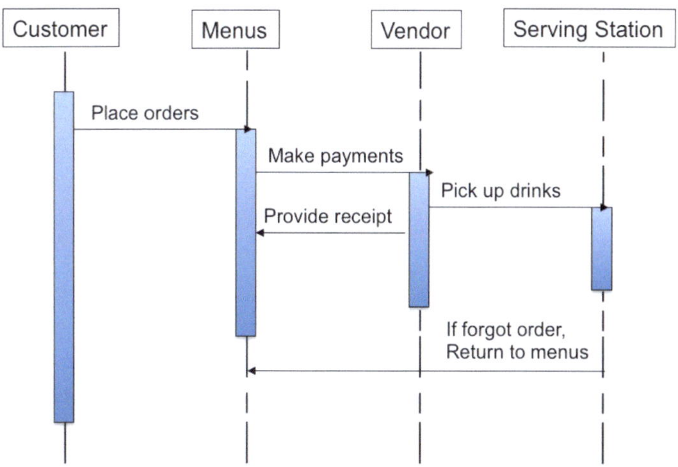

FIG. 5 Sequence of events diagram

organization's value proposition? In the lemonade stand example, this could be timely delivery of low calorie-content lemonade juice.

- Implement *Kanban* (meaning signboard or billboard in Japanese). This is a scheduling system for lean and just-in-time operation used in production. The idea here is to avoid wastes via real-time demand signaling across the supply chain and to align demand with supply. Keeping an active updated inventory enables production of the right amount of service at the right time [4]. In the lemonade stand example, this means factoring in seasonal changes in the supply of lemons to match and meet high demand in seasons like the summer.
- Set up spaghetti diagrams (Fig. 6 and Table 7).

(iv)**Standards:** The following components must be considered when establishing standards for the process at hand [5].

- Internal standards: Establish uniform standards across the organization at the macro- and micro-

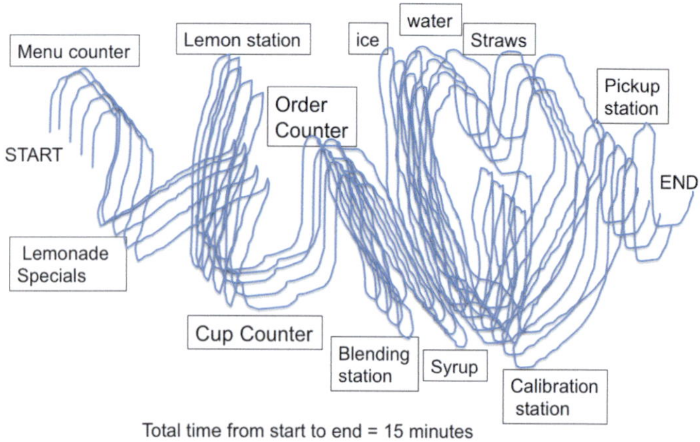

Fig. 6 Spaghetti diagram

TABLE 7 Spaghetti diagram

What does this do? Sets up a visual layout of workflow and maps out the actual flow of movement from one unit to the next. It is helpful in lean process mapping to identify bottlenecks and inefficiencies to geographical movement
How does it work?
Spatially identifies areas that are too distant and result in unnecessary and inefficient movement and helps staff to decide which areas to bring together to optimize work flow and movement. For example, this helps eliminate wasteful transportation cost and time

levels. Using the lemonade stand, for example, all lemonade drinks must have on the average 2 % sugar content with acceptable 0.05 % variance; all vendors must use the same menus and prioritize timely service delivery.

- Outside standards: Have consistent standards that satisfy demands of the external environment. Say, for example, that the FDA requires that the lemonade contains at least 10 % lemon juice. This is a standard set by an outside governing body, for instance, all the lemonade stands in your neighborhood have on the average 12 % lemon juice content, which is a standard by other peoples' performance, and the lemonade business must try to meet this outside standard.
- Voice of the customer: Must be central to all aspects of planning and QI implementation, for example, taking customer feedback to improve the service, especially cutting down on customer wait times, or providing variety of lemonade specialized according to customer demands.
- Stakeholder analysis template: Engage leadership and management to safeguard feasibility and support for the project. Identify and communicate early with key people to establish common goals and consensus. In the lemonade stand business, potential stakehold-

ers will include: (1) shareholders or joint owners of the business (who may have financial standards for profit margins and may only want to be in business if profit margin exceeds a particular threshold), (2) lemonade vendors (who may expect steady work hours), (3) lemon suppliers (who may expect certain level of demand and will not provide lemon supply below some threshold), (4) neighbors in the location of the business (who have to deal with lots of people standing in line for lemonade creating noise), and (5) other lemonade competitors (who want you out of the business) [2, 6].

2. **Prioritize the problem:**

   - CTQ, meaning critical to quality: Identify the parameters that are important to provide quality product or service, for example, regular tune-up of lemonade blenders for making the lemon juice.
   - Key performance indicators: Establishing a priori quantifiable markers of success will allow for goal-oriented solutions, for example, cutting down wait times by 50 % and increasing sales by 25 %.
   - Stakeholder analysis: Prioritize the problems based on stakeholder input and support, for example, taking customer feedback seriously to implement changes in the sugar content of lemonade and providing workers more time off.

3. **Types of things to measure:** Ask "what does better look like?" and measure parameters that show improvement. This may be qualitative or quantitative. Measurements may focus on improvements in outcomes (lemonade which is not too sweet or too sour consistently, with parameters, e.g., 20 % sugar content with 1 % acceptable variance), structure (better working environment where people don't trip on wires, have windows to look out of, have water fountains accessible, etc.; again, this can be measured using number of wires that can be tripped on, percentage improvement in windows per cubicle, etc.), or processes

(improved variance, e.g., cut down variance from 10 % of average to 3 % of average, decreased wait time, decreased non-value added time, decreased waste, e.g., 10 % less wrappers to throw out, 20 % less defective lemonade cups produced, etc.). See spaghetti diagram Fig. 6 for a qualitative improvement example of showing how reorganizing spatial workflow will likely decrease customer wait times and is an example of reorganizing the structure to affect process outcomes.

4. **Define problem scope:** Understand the boundaries and limitations of the project as well as time and resource constraints. For example, hiring more customer service personnel may speed up service, but this comes at cost for the lemonade stand business. This limitation could be alternatively addressed via spatial workflow rearrangement. As shown in Fig. 6, if the goal is to improve service at one location to satisfy a certain class of customers who are willing to pay more for quicker services, one may hire more personnel at one location and test run it as a deluxe service (i.e., to compare to the regular slow service) to see how this changes the services.
5. **Plan the change and set goals:**

    - Obtain team buy-in. For example, rally all customer service personnel to provide input regarding workflow reorganization and to work together toward improving service delivery. Say, for example, based on prior stakeholder analysis, one knows that the business owners want more profit margins, while the workers and staff want a safer work environment; it may be easier to persuade staff that by making the appropriate changes to decrease customer wait time, there would be more profit margins for the business and workers could get bonuses, have less clutter for accidents hence a safer environment, or have less things to clean up after work enabling them to leave work earlier.
    - Team culture: Establish culture with quality values and QI philosophy. For example, all lemonade vendors prioritize high customer service and feedback.

- Set good effective goals and prepare the team to facilitate change acceptance. For example, in the lemonade stand business, an effective and specific goal would be cutting down delivery time by 25 % by the end of the summer sales period.

6. **Error proofing:** Also known as the poka-yoke (pronounced as "poh-kah yoh-kay"). The goal is to eliminate errors and reduce waste. Set up fail-safe mechanisms and empower all team members to adopt a fail-safe mindset, for example, having an automatic glucometer off-switch system installed within all the lemonade mixing blenders such that the blenders have an alarm beep that goes off if the percentage of sugar content is above or below a preset concentration [7].
7. **Make team decisions:**

- Brainstorming – usually performed as a group activity. The group meets to write down ideas about addressing issues or topic of interest on notes cards and mount on a board display. Brainstorming facilitates team work and helps open discussions about projects.
- Cost-benefit matrix – identify all the positive and negative factors and quantify the anticipated financial revenue to help prioritize which projects to tackle first, i.e., high-impact, low-cost projects (Fig. 7 and Table 8). In

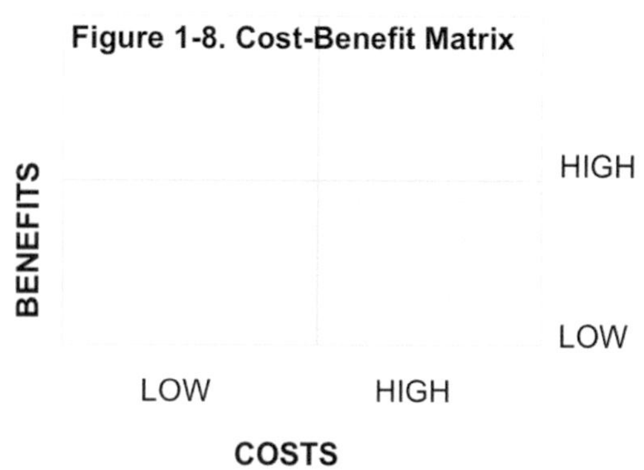

FIG. 7 Cost-benefit matrix

Table 8 Cost-benefit matrix
What does this do? Sets up a matrix outlining high vs. low end-value generating projects. Enables cost-effective allocation of resources
How does it work? This is a simple foursquare map (two-by-two table) that visually lays out the anticipated impact of a project on the vertical axis and the associated financial value and costs on the horizontal axis. Helps to prioritize initiatives in order of highest to lowest impact vs. cost

the lemonade stand example, a high-impact, low-cost project would be reducing wait times by having dispensers that can deliver made-to-order amounts of lemonade per customer; so rather than waiting in line, customers are given cups as soon as they order, so they can self-serve from the dispenser, rather than wait in line. Usually, low-cost, high-benefit options are sought after first, and if they are not available, cost-benefit analysis would be performed, e.g., it's worth it for the business to buy expansive dispensers to keep the business running, rather than continue to have high variability in lemonade and go out of business.

8. **Assign jobs:**

   - Define roles and responsibilities using the RACI (responsible, accountable, consulted, informed) chart (Table 9) [8]. In the lemonade stand business, assign personnel to the menu station, ingredient station, delivery station, and payment stations.

- Key roles to assign for a quality improvement project prior to undertaking the project: Team leader (e.g., lemonade business owners), team members (lemon suppliers, vendors, and salesmen), subject matter experts (connoisseur and world lemonade expert), champion (proud neighborhood, lemonade drink supporter, and nutritionists), process owner (waiters, mixer, and servers), and master black

Table 9 RACI chart

R: *Responsible*
Who is or will be doing the task?
Who has been assigned to work on the task?
A: *Accountable*
Who is in charge of the project?
Who answers when things go wrong?
C: *Consulted*
Who are the experts to be consulted?
I: *Informed*
Who needs to be updated regarding the progress of the project?

belts (highly trained experts in the use of Six Sigma processing and analytic tools to address quality problems).

9. **Generate a lean A3 diagram:** A3 (refers to A3-size paper) is a tool used for lean design. This tool helps with performing root cause analysis by reducing your problem to its core on one page of paper. This lean approach to addressing problems is centered on Kaizen (a Japanese term for continuous and consistent improvement); it helps to eliminate non-value-adding processes [9]. A3 pools together all the previous tools – process flowchart, fishbone diagram, etc. – for problem solving (Table 10). More discussion on lean and lean processes follows in the next session.

Table 10 A3 template

Problem statement: In one or two sentences, briefly state the problem and its symptoms. For example, customers wait too long in line for lemonade
Background and current state of affairs: Where are the gaps in performance? Quantify and describe the patterns of occurrence of the problem. What are the conditions and parameters? For example, workstations have poor spatial arrangement leading to superfluous movement from one station to the next
Root cause analysis: Ask the five whys. Why does the problem exist? Break down each reason or cause until further breakdown is impossible. Distinguish the underlying reason (real) vs. apparent or contributing symptoms. For example, why are wait times long? Because stations are not well organized. Why are the stations not well organized? And so on and so forth
Goals and metrics: What outcomes should be anticipated from resolution of the identified problem? How would you measure improvements? For example, reorganizing workstations should increase workflow and decrease customer wait times. Measure the cycle time for lemonade production and delivery (from order to pick up) and customer satisfaction surveys
Scope: Define what will be retained vs. what will be eliminated. For example, eliminate cup counters and retain the supply station
Proposed countermeasures: Evaluate possible solutions based on cost, time to implement, and effectiveness of the solutions. For example, reorganizing workstations and hiring more personnel to run the stations
Timeline: Establish project completion date. For example, project to be completed by summer sales quarter

Do

- Execute and implement the change on a **small scale**:

  1. Process

(a) Redesign the process.
(b) Task share.
(c) Increase staff.
(d) Reduce waste.
(e) Minimize variability by standardizing.
(f) Kaizen approach: Perform continuous and consistent improvement.
(g) Apply one-piece rather than batch-flow processing [10]. The former tackles a single item at a time to precisely meet customer pull and avoids unnecessary buildup, allows for efficient customization, and yields better quality products. The latter, batch processing, builds up an inventory of parts before starting production. This tends to lead to waste given the volume and variability of customer demands. Batching leads to more waiting and downtime and increased rework and delays when a defect is discovered in an entire batch rather than in a single unit.

2. Structure

(a) Organize structure by 5S checklist: sort, set in order, shine, standardize, and sustain.
(b) As discussed before, Kanban (signal to perform work) should be part of this phase of the PDCA. Kanban allows supply chain to respond quickly and specifically to customer demand.
(c) Line layout: organize workstations according to activities being performed. Workstations facilitate high-volume output [11]. Drawing from the lemonade stand example, having a mixing station for lemonade vs. a lemon-squeezing station vs. a dispensing station helps to increase economies of scale by allowing individual processes to function more efficiently.

- Apply lean and Six Sigma principles of change: The **term lean production was** first used by John Krafcik to describe the Japanese Toyota Manufacturing and Production

System [12]. The goal of lean methodology is waste reduction and elimination by streamlining processes that use up resources but generate no value. Lean applies to both product manufacturing and processes; it is a way of thinking that holds relevance for every industry from healthcare to manufacturing to education. The underlying idea is to foster smooth flow, making the right product at the right time in the right amounts for the right customer. This dates back to 1913, in Highland Park, Michigan, with the Ford Automobile. Henry Ford pioneered flow production when he designed fabrication sequence production for automobiles. Using go and no-go gauges, his company was able to fabricate and assemble automobile components into perfectly fit ready-to-drive vehicles within minutes. However, this system of production was unable to provide customized vehicles and variety to meet consumer needs. His methods worked great in a steady state environment, but began to fall short in a dynamic environment with uncertain and constant changes. In the 1930s, Kiichiro Toyoda, Taiichi Ohno, and others at Toyota developed the Total Production System, as a revised improvement of Ford's assembly line production system [13]. Toyota production system was centered around Kaizen (improvement) teams with emphasis on the smooth product flow through the total manufacturing process. The goal was to establish value-adding processes at all steps of production and cut down on the time and information needed to meet the customer's needs. They identified three types of wastes: *muri*, *mura*, and *muda*. Muri refers to excessiveness/unreasonableness/over-burden and it can be eliminated by standardization. Mura refers to unevenness or irregularity and can be eliminated by the just-in-time approach to production. For example, when a defect is identified in one process, the problem is identified and corrected immediately before moving on to the next step. Muda refers to futility and can be eliminated by focusing on enhancing value-adding work and cutting down on non-value-adding work. While muri and mura need to be addressed in lean production, this chapter will limit its discussion to mudas, of which there are seven common ones [14].

- Identify and tackle the seven mudas: transportation, inventory, motion, waiting, over-processing, overproduction, and defects. In the lemonade stand example, waste of transportation would be separate shipment of lemonade ingredient batches to vendors; waste of inventory will be stocking ingredients without a forecast of demand; waste of motion would be the redundancy of separating out the steps of squeezing lemons from blending lemon juice and filtering lemon seeds (Remember motion = moving of people, transport = moving items); waste of waiting would refer to the extra time customers have to wait in line; waste of over-processing would be manually serving lemonade vs. using a dispensing machine to serve; waste of overproduction would refer to making more lemonade than is required; and defects would refer to lack of standardization about mixing ratios of lemon juice to sugar to water mix.
- Practice pull-type rather than push-type processes. In pull-type processing, production is based on the level of demand. Thus, products can be custom-made and designed to meet consumer needs (also known as just-in-time processing). In push-type processing, production is not based on demand. Rather, product supply continues to happen independent of the demand and extra products stored in the inventory.
- Stop when a mistake happens and try to devise a solution before moving to the next step. Keep work processes transparent, allow room to stop, check and correct errors, and empower frontline workers to control the process.
- Match Takt and cycle times. In simple terms, Takt time refers to the ratio of the time available to complete a project that provides value and the average demand within that time frame. Takt = [Available Time / Average Demand]. For example, if the highest demand for lemonade is between 12 noon and 1 p.m. and within that hour, there are 20 customers waiting in line, then the Takt time = 60 min / 20 = 3. This

means that every 3 min a customer would be requesting a cup of lemonade, and to meet just-in-time demand, lemonade has to be served every 3 min. For the cycle time, let's say it takes Jane Doe (who is the waitress at the counter) an average of 1 min to take the order, and it takes John Smith (the waiter making the lemonade) an average of 2 min to finish and serve the lemonade, and then the cycle time for ready-to-serve lemonade, from the time the order is taken, would be 3 min if these are the only two participants in the process of lemonade delivery to the customer after the order was taken. Cycle time refers to the lowest repeatable time to produce the finished product. Ideally Takt and cycle times should match perfectly as in this hypothetical lemonade stand example to avoid wasted time of customers waiting in line. In practice, it's often customary to take into account inefficiencies of the system and allow for say 10–20 % lag in the cycle time to match real-life takt time demands. Typically Takt and cycle times are synced in scenarios requiring repetitive tasks that have predictable demand. When Takt and cycle times do not match, it is instructive to find out the sources of processing inefficiencies and tackle them.

- In contrast to lean methodology, the main philosophy of Six Sigma is error reduction and minimization of variability. The goal is to produce a level of product quality within six standard deviations from average (an error rate of about 0.0003 % or an accuracy rate of 99.9996 %). Six Sigma focuses on customer value and employs DMAIC as one of its analytic tools (see previous chapter discussion, Box 1). Standardize processes and material supplies.
- Use clearly defined SOE diagrams (Table 6, and Fig. 5) and spaghetti diagrams (Fig. 6) for workflow specifications to minimize variability.
- Create habitual work performance standards, for example, all lemonade business personnel incentivized to be invested in timely delivery of lemonade.

Check/Study

During this phase of the project, the QI team members should stop to evaluate the progress in the process improvement. Try to figure out what has changed and see what the group has learned. How can the lessons be applied on a small scale? Apply the tools previously discussed in the reevaluation process: fishbone diagrams (Fig. 3), spaghetti diagram (Fig. 6), value stream map (Table 5), and root cause analysis (Table 10). To be clear, at up to this point in the process, change is being implemented on a small scale, for example, focusing on only one lemonade stand and its spatial reorganization. At the *checkpoint*, the QI team evaluates the interventions and their effects are produced on the small scale. This is in preparation for the next step in the cycle, which is the ACT phase, where one attempts to expand the small experiment to the larger scale.

Act (and Also Control)

- Execute on a larger scale and resume the cycle, for example, reorganizing all lemonade stand workstations across the city to have the same setup and using the model from the initial test site.
- Create buy-in, for example, talking to all suppliers of lemons and blending machines, customers, sales agents, and vendors to confirm that everyone is on the same page regarding reorganizing the lemonade workstations.
- Apply ten rules of Kaizen (continuous improvement, elimination of waste); see Box 1.
- Reassess priorities based on what was learned in check/study phase by performing a cost-benefit matrix (Table 8).
- Create a sustainable system of implementation, e.g., using Six Sigma to monitor the process variability. For example, require all lemonade businesses to have three key workstations organized to increase work flow (see Fig. 5).

- If goals are achieved, start controlling.
    1. Document the improved process and make sure it's being followed. For example, what is the lemonade cycle time? Is it matching up with the Takt time? Are customers spending less waiting in line for lemonade?
    2. Implement mistake-proofing tools – poka-yoke; see if functioning, for example, verifying percentage of sugar content of lemonade with calibrator at the blending station and adjusting percent concentration before moving to the dispensing phase.
    3. Control plan – what key metrics/processes need to be documented to make sure gains are sustained? Control plan template.

Box 1: The Ten Rules of Kaizen

Kaizen is a Japanese word, which means gradual and continuous change. It is a central theme of lean thinking and philosophy. The idea is to improve processes by cutting out non-value-adding processes. The principles of Kaizen are as outlined with examples:

- ***Question convention:*** *look for new better ways.* For example, conventional wisdom suggests that if one is sick, especially if one is hospitalized, one should be resting in bed. However, with one or two exceptions, this is not exactly correct. Hazards of bed rest and inactivity include debility, cardiopulmonary and functional decline, increased risk of venous thromboembolism, and pressure ulcers.
- ***Solve problems:*** *think of how to improve the status quo, not why things cannot change*. For example, one way to minimize inactivity and unnecessary bed rest is to monitor and measure patient mobility with the HAL (highest activity level) scale.
- ***Collect data, test assumptions:*** For example, do patients with high activity scores develop better hospital outcomes than those with low scores?

- ***Fix errors now, not later:*** For example, for wrong-limb surgery, create a checklist and time-out process to prevent future mistakes.
- **Set SMART goals and standards:** For example, decrease pressure ulcers related to bed immobility by 20 % in 6 months. Set unit-wide compliance target rates. SMART goals refer to specific, measurable, attainable, realistic, and timely. SMART goals help set specific targets and have higher likelihood of being accomplished than generic non-SMART goals.
- ***Work efficiently, smarter, not harder:*** For example, recruit frontline staff such as nursing to implement and monitor out-of-bed activities for patients.
- ***Collate group wisdom, not money*:** To solve problems, gather group consensus first; money is a secondary matter. For example, conduct surveys of medical team to identify barriers to patient functional mobility, generate ideas for solutions, and discuss feasibility of proposed solutions.
- ***Target root causes:*** For example, why are patient getting unnecessary bed rests? Is it due to lack of knowledge of the associated risks? Is it a problem of understaffing?
- ***Lead by example:*** Be an enabler. Encourage and recognize frontline staff for their efforts and contributions.
- ***Work in teams:*** A multidisciplinary approach to problem solving yields better results than a singular approach.

References

1. Donabedian A. The methods and findings of quality assessment and monitoring: an illustrated analysis. Ann Arbor: Health Administration Press; 1985.
2. Huson M, Nanda D. The impact of just-in-time manufacturing on firm performance in the US. J Oper Manage. 1995;12(3):297–310.
3. Michalska J, Szewieczek D. The 5S methodology as a tool for improving the organization. J Achiev Mater Manuf Eng. 2007;24(2):211–4.
4. Anderson DJ. Kanban. Blue Hole Press, Seattle, Washington, ISBN-10: 0984521402, 2010.

5. Ghobadian A, Speller S, Jones M. Service quality: concepts and models. Int J Qual Reliab Manage. 1994;11(9):43–66.
6. Hyder A, Syed S, Puvanachandra P, Bloom G, Sundaram S, Mahmood S, et al. Stakeholder analysis for health research: case studies from low-and middle-income countries. Public Health. 2010;124(3):159–66.
7. Varkey P, Reller MK, Resar RK. Basics of quality improvement in health care. Mayo Clinic Proceedings; Elsevier; 2007.
8. Johnson M, Capasso V. Improving patient flow through the emergency department. J Healthcare Manage. 2012;57(4):236–43.
9. Jimmerson C, Weber D, Sobek DK. Reducing waste and errors: piloting lean principles at Intermountain Healthcare. Jt Comm J Qual Patient Saf. 2005;31(5):249–57.
10. Burbidge JL. The" new approach" to production. Prod Engineer. 1961;40(12):769–84.
11. Burbidge JL. Production flow analysis. Prod Engineer. 1971;50(4.5):139–52.
12. Aycock J. A brief history of just-in-time. ACM Comput Surv (CSUR). 2003;35(2):97–113.
13. Sugimori Y, Kusunoki K, Cho F, Uchikawa S. Toyota production system and kanban system materialization of just-in-time and respect-for-human system. Int J Prod Res. 1977;15(6):553–64.
14. Wittenberg G. Kaizen—the many ways of getting better. Assem Autom. 1994;14(4):12–7.

Lean Sigma Case Study

Richard Hill

> **Tools**
> A3, balance arrow, benefit effort matrix, control chart, fishbone diagram, Kanban, SIPOC, spaghetti diagram, value stream map, waste walk

Background

Kate was very excited to be hired as the operations manager for a busy pediatric practice. In this role, she is responsible for the coordination of four physicians, two physician assistants, two nurses, and two office staff. Kate brought extensive experience gained from being the office manager of a smaller practice so she felt comfortable in accepting this new position. It did not take long, however, for her to realize that there were significant scheduling, throughput, and patient-related issues which she tried unsuccessfully to address.

R. Hill (✉)
Armstrong Institute for Patient Safety and Quality,
Johns Hopkins Medicine, 750 East Pratt Street, 15th Floor,
Baltimore, MD 21202, USA
e-mail: rhill26@jhmi.edu

L. Atanelov (ed.), *Resident's Handbook of Medical Quality and Safety*, DOI 10.1007/978-3-319-24190-6_30

Kate's brother, Howard, called at the end of a particularly bad day, and Kate confided that she was at a loss to be able to fix the various problems and was seriously thinking about quitting. Howard asked if she would share the issues in detail with him. Listening intently and asking periodic questions, Howard suggested that she hold off on quitting for the time being as perhaps this was a "process" issue that could be fixed. It turns out that he was a certified Lean Sigma Black Belt so indeed; he knew a thing or two about processes. Howard agreed to take a week off from work to help her out. They agreed to start 3 weeks later on Monday and that Kate would talk to the staff and explain that her brother was going to offer "free" consulting help. All that was needed from the staff was 2 h per day to contribute their expertise in a facilitated team setting. This process would typically occur over a period of weeks, but this would need to be a rapid improvement event (RIE) in which a project is done in an accelerated period of time.

Gemba

The place where the work is done.

Howard arrived on Monday about a half hour before the patients arrived. He explained that the first step would be for him to go to the gemba, watch, and take notes. He told Kate that it is critical to watch what happens there in order to see the "real truth" vs. what is "thought" to happen.

A3

A one-page document that documents the work being done and what needs to happen next.

After observing for several hours, Howard pulled an 11 × 16 in. piece of paper from his briefcase. He explained that the document is called an A3 problem-solving tool. Its purpose he explained is to document the baseline process and employ the scientific method to develop an improved and sustainable process. The idea is that the document at any point in time should reflect the work being done at whatever stage the process it's in. The format varies; however, it typically uses the PDCA (plan, do, check, act) or DMAIC (define, measure, analyze, improve, control) format (Fig. 1).

The first items to be listed on the A3 are the statement of the problem, followed by a goal, metric, and team composition. After some conversation, they agreed on the following and entered it on the A3.

Define (DMAIC) or Plan (PDCA) Phase

Problem

Patient visit times are unpredictable and lengthy resulting in patient and staff dissatisfaction potentially leading to a loss of patients and employee turnover.

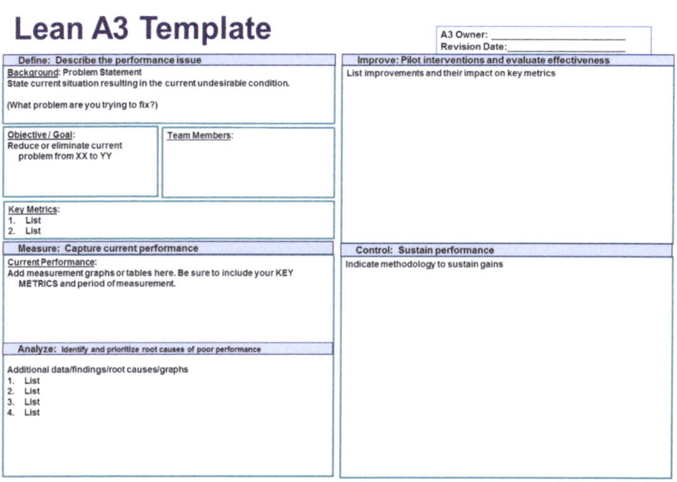

FIG. 1 Lean A3 template

Goal

Reduce the patient's average lead (throughput) time from XX to YY minutes (20 % reduction) by December 31.

Metric

Big Y = Average throughput time in minutes for patient visits (excluding new patient visits) and limited to weekday hours only (see Scope section on page XX).

Kate's next step was to collect data on the length of patient visits over the past 2 months in order to determine what the actual baseline and 20 % reduction would equate to.

Team

All staff members (small size and the need for all to participate).

Measure (DMAIC) or Plan (PDCA) Phase

Baseline Data

The "as is" state of the process.

Early the next day, Kate was able to obtain the additional baseline patient data for the past 2 months. She provided a spreadsheet file with the following information in columns: patient #, visit date, appt. time, sign-in time, departure time, chief complaint, provider, and procedure.

Howard downloaded this information on his laptop and began to "crunch the data." The first order of business was to use the data to add specificity to the project goal. He calculated the mean (mathematical average) as 114 min. Since the goal was a 20 % reduction over the mean and it appears to be reasonable, the goal statement was changed as follows:

Revised Goal

Reduce the patient's average lead time (throughput) from **114 to 91** min (20 % reduction) by December 31.

Sampling

Obtaining partial data representative of the population.

Since we do not have data for all clinic visits, we are working with a sample. It is important that our sample is representative:

- Composition – reflects the larger population in terms of composition and contains little bias.
- Size – enough data points to ensure meaningful analysis and interpretation is possible. In general a minimum of 30 points for variable data and 100 points for attribute data – more is better but weigh cost vs. benefit of obtaining the data:
- **Attribute/categorical data** – Can be placed in a discrete category – e.g., yes/no, hot/cold, good/bad, and limited choices such as a five-point pain scale.
- **Variables/continuous data** – On a continuum, can be meaningfully be subdivided into smaller units of measure, e.g., volume, temperature, time, and weight.

Measurement Systems Analysis (MSA)

An assessment of the adequacy of the measurement system:

- Seeks to reduce variation in the measurement system:
  - Establish an operational definition of each data collected – who is measuring, how is it to be measured, using what tools, and when is it collected.
  - For example, lead time is measured from the time the patient is registered until the patient leaves the clinic as measured by the registration staff using the wall clock.

- Must validate the data to ensure it is accurate and in adherence to the operational definition.
- Ensure the process is **repeatable** (one person uses the same process and gets the same result for the same thing measured) and **reproducible** (multiple people using the same process obtain the same result each time for the same thing being measured):

We have included all providers working on weekdays within the last 2 months so the data is representative of the larger population (all data). There were complete data for 1374 patient encounters out of a total of 2122 patient encounters over the past 2 months. The differences in the data are that not all included the patient's departure time. Since there was no pattern in the uncaptured departure times, we could conclude that these were random events and not subject to bias.

Several audits were conducted to review the process and determine if the lead time is accurately reflected by the registration staff. The data were deemed to be accurate and fit for use.

Data Stability

The predictability of data to fall within a range demonstrating minimal volatility.

Control Chart

A tool to assess stability, help see variation, detect changes, and see patterns over time (Fig. 2).

- Data points must be in time series order.
- The area between the upper and lower control limits establishes the normal range of variation.
- Control limits are determined by the process – typically 3 standard deviations above and below the mean.

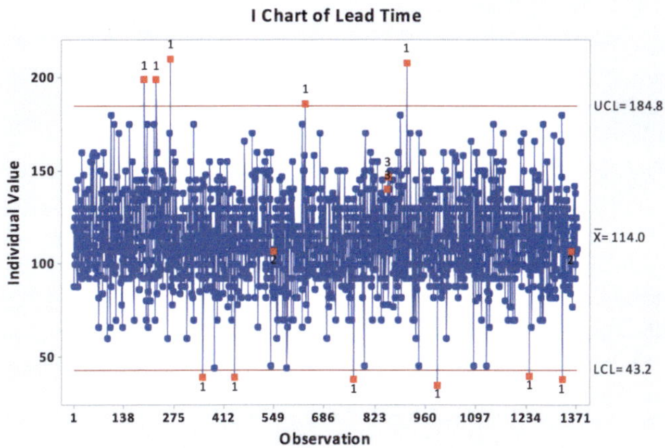

FIG. 2 Individual's control chart

- Points below the lower control limits/above the upper control limits are typically due to special cause variation, i.e., something unusual, <1 % chance; it happens by chance alone in normal data.
- A process is said to be in control and the data is usable if:
- Ninety-five percent of the points are between the lower and upper control limits.
- No significant trends (six or more consecutive points increasing or decreasing).
- No significant shifts (nine or more consecutive points above or below the center line (mean)).
- If any of the above special causes exists, they must first be identified for cause.

Our control chart demonstrated few special causes out of the total number of data points so we could conclude that our data passes the test and is therefore usable for analysis.

Lean Metrics

Value Stream Map (VSM)

High-level depiction of a process with connected process steps, system interactions, and time elements.

"This picture represents our process," said Howard. Steps that have a triangle preceding it represent the time the patient was waiting to begin the step. Each step and wait time is labeled with a time in minutes. This completed map is typically added to the A3 to visualize the process.

He then drew in red the various metrics and their meanings. See Fig. 3.

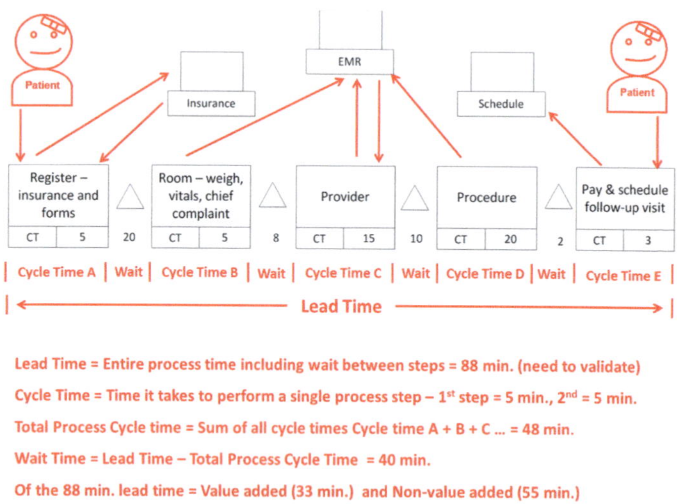

Fig. 3 Clinic value stream map

Analyze (DMAIC) or Plan (PDCA) Phase

Howard outlined his takeaways from the information:

- The longest step called the constraint step is the procedure – this step controls the pace of the line, but this only happens about 30 % of the time. The provider piece is the 2nd longest and happens 100 % of the time.
- The longest wait time is between the register and in the room (20 min) because the rooms are all typically full.
- The EMR is the most frequently used "data system" – used in 3 steps.

Kate asked, "How can you be so sure that these times are correct based on 1 day's observation?" Howard explained that the VSM data only needs to be "directionally correct" and that precision is not required. "We are simply trying to see where the opportunity is in using this tool," he explained. Our largest area of opportunity in this case will be minimizing the time waiting between steps.

Value Add/Non-Value Add (VA/NVA)

All time as shown on the map can be broken down into two categories, value added and non-value added. This is in the "eyes of your customer." If you provided a customer with a detailed bill with every activity listed, what would they pay for? The items chosen would be value-added activities and the rest non-value added.

Value added (VA) = lead (throughput) time minus NVA (what the customer feels is valuable):

Example: (88 min LT) – (55 min NVA) = 33 min VA

Non-value added (NVA) = lead (throughput) time minus VA (customer is not willing to pay for):

Example: (88 LT min) – (33 min VA) = 55 min NVA

Howard explained that the goal of the value added is to decrease it further if it makes sense, but the real opportunity is to eliminate as much NVA as possible. Kate thought about it and asked, "Some value added is necessary even if the patient doesn't think so, right?" That is true, there is one more category of value called the necessary non-value added (NNVA). These are the items that are non-value added but we absolutely need to do in order to provide our service. All of the seven wastes are NVA.

Necessary non-value added (NNVA) – (subset of NVA that we **must** do), e.g., double check for safety:

Example: Of the 55 min of NVA, only 5 min of which was considered necessary – this was the time the patient waited in the room for the provider to enter his notes in the system.

Ideally you should ask your patients directly as to which category each activity belongs, but as a surrogate, you can ask your staff to determine this as if a loved one was a patient going through a visit.

Voice of the Customer (VOC)

Critical needs and wants of the customer.

Many times we just assume we know what is acceptable to our customers, but what if we are not correct? What is an acceptable visit length? We need to ask our patients. Perhaps we can survey them. While we are at it, we can ask them other questions such as what is important to them about their visit. We can then ensure we are meeting their needs or not making something worse with our new process.

SIPOC

(see chapter discussing topic) Howard explained the tool to Kate and they drafted one together. "We can have the team finish it up tomorrow," said Howard. The suppliers and customers will help us determine if we have the right team composition, and the inputs and outputs will provide additional information about contributors to long appointment times and variation.

Takt Time [1]

The rate the process needs to meet or exceed in order to keep up with demand: the "heartbeat."

Another question that we need to ask is how well is our process working – are we keeping up with our patient load throughout the day or do we fall behind? Kate said, "We don't do so well, many of us never have time to take a lunch because we are so busy." The following formula may be applied to provide an objective answer:

Takt time = Available work time/demand

Example: The office staff work 8 h and we see patients for 7.5 h. We saw a total of 2,122 patients over a 40-day period which equates to 53 patients per day.

Available work time = 7.5 h × 60 min = 450 min

Demand = 53 patients, and takt time = 450 min/53 patients = 8.5 min per patient

The practical significance of this is that in order to keep up with demand, we must discharge a patient every 8.5 min or less; otherwise we fall behind and play "catch up" working longer hours. Any process step-cycle time exceeding the 8.5 min takt time will prohibit us from keeping up with demand. Refer to the preceding VSM. Note that the provider time (15 minutes) and procedure time (20 minutes) both exceed the takt time. These two steps should now be targeted for additional focus.

Balance Arrow

Tool to analyze and show VA/NVA/NNVA cycle time components and comparison of each to takt (Fig. 4).

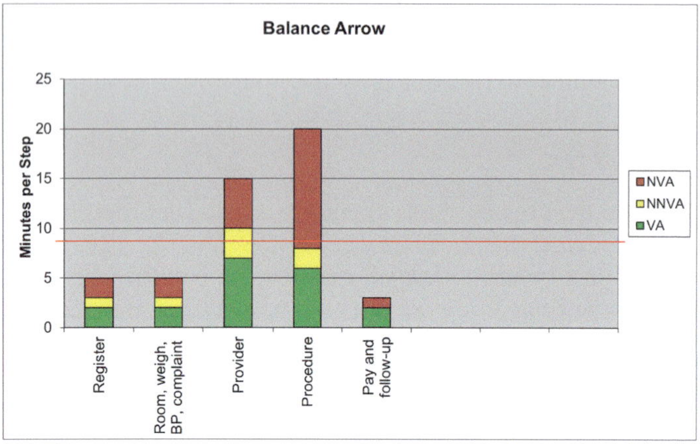

FIG. 4 Clinic cycle time balance arrow

The balance arrow is constructed by the team:

- Focus is on the cycle times that exceed takt.
- Detail level steps are identified with approximate times assigned to each.
- Each time per category is summed and the stacked bar is created.
- VA (green) is on the bottom, NNVA (yellow) in the middle, and NVA (red) on top.

The finished chart illustrates that there is an opportunity to improve the two steps exceeding takt, due to the amount of NVA contained in each.

Spaghetti Map

A "rough" scale drawing of the gemba layout tracing the flow of work.

Howard and Kate drew the layout of the clinic on a flip chart. They then observed several patient encounters, tracing the flow. See Fig. 5.

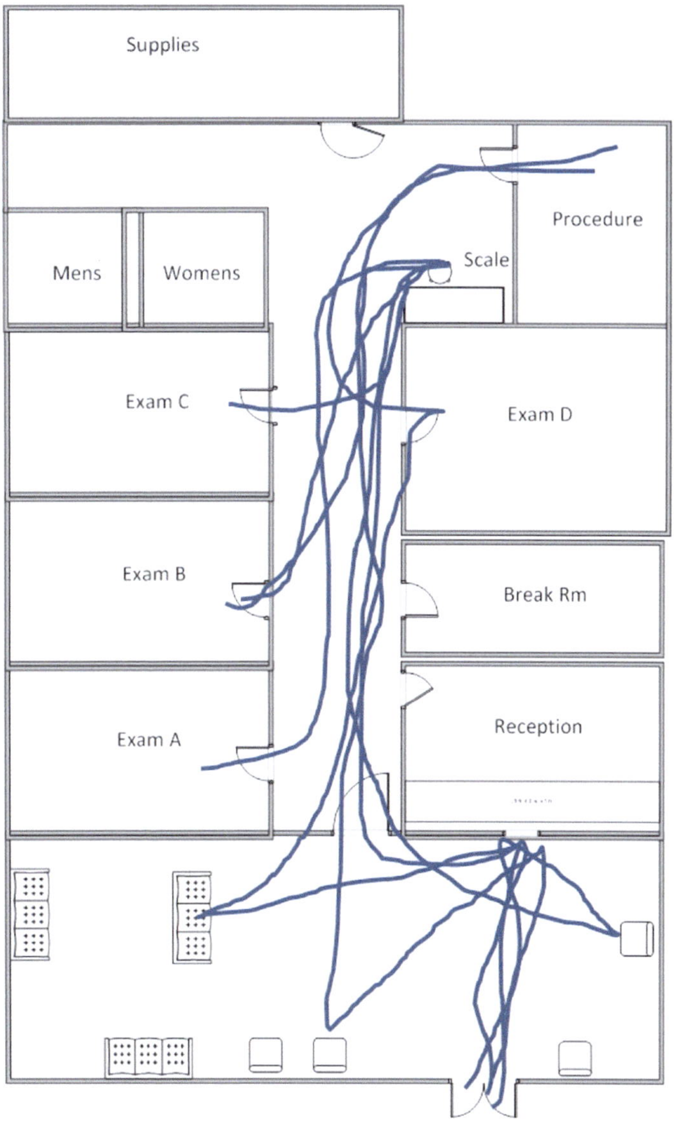

FIG. 5 Spaghetti map of clinic flow

Every patient needs to be weighed. The scale is located in the back of the clinic. In addition, the break room is in the front of the clinic taking up "prime real estate."

Team

It was now time to meet as a team for the first meeting represented by all critical parties – the physicians, PAs, nursing, and administrative staff. The agenda items were as follows:

1. Discuss the imperative – What problem are we trying to fix and why?
2. Review Lean Sigma basic principles – What is Lean, Six Sigma, and DMAIC.
3. Review the A3 as completed to date.
4. Complete the SIPOC for missed items.
5. Review the spaghetti map.
6. Review the seven wastes in preparation for the "waste walk."

Waste Walk

Team activity to go to the gemba and observe the process step-by-step in order to see and categorize the non-value-added activities (waste).

The Seven Process Wastes

1. Defects – undesirable things that require rework to fix, e.g., missing documentation
2. Overproduction – making too many of something, e.g., scheduling too many patients
3. Motion – of the staff, e.g., leaving the room to get supplies
4. Overprocessing – doing unnecessary work, e.g., ordering unnecessary tests
5. Waiting – staff, patients, and families, e.g., waiting in rooms, waiting for provider, etc.

6. Inventory – too much, too little, and wrong location, e.g., sorting to find what's needed
7. Transportation – movement of the "thing" in the process, e.g., patient moves to be weighed

Waste Walk Steps

1. Each team member was handed sticky notes and a fine tip marker.
2. The entire team went to the gemba and pulled a file of a patient. Howard pretended he was that patient going step-by-step through the process.
3. Each member was allowed to ask questions to better understand the process as it was happening.
4. Each member individually wrote down one waste per post it noted.
5. Upon completion, Howard asked one person at a time to read their note and place it on the wall by the appropriate process step as listed on the SIPOC.

A total of 68 waste notes were now on the wall. Now, the team was given a different color of sticky notes and asked to write a potential solution for each. These were then read aloud and stuck on the wall with the appropriate waste. A total of 26 potential solutions were suggested.

Benefit Effort Matrix

This tool is used to prioritize potential interventions based on the level of benefit derived vs. the level of effort required to launch it.

Benefit

The level of favorable impact on your Big Y (key metric)

Effort

Time, expense, and involvement of resources

The matrix is drawn on a flip chart and each of the "sticky-note" solutions are placed in the appropriate area as determined by the team. The matrix is constructed per the following (Fig. 6):

Out of the 26 items, 6 were in the first quadrant, 3 were in the second, 10 were in the third, and 7 were in the fourth. These interventions (all in quadrant one) were selected.

- Move the weight scale to the registration area from the end of the hall, reducing motion/transportation, and have the registration person weigh and record, reducing nurse workload.
- Swap the break room with the procedure room – motion and transportation.
- Determine additional medical record input nursing could do – reduce MD/PA room time.
- Stock room with additional frequently used supplies – reduce motion.

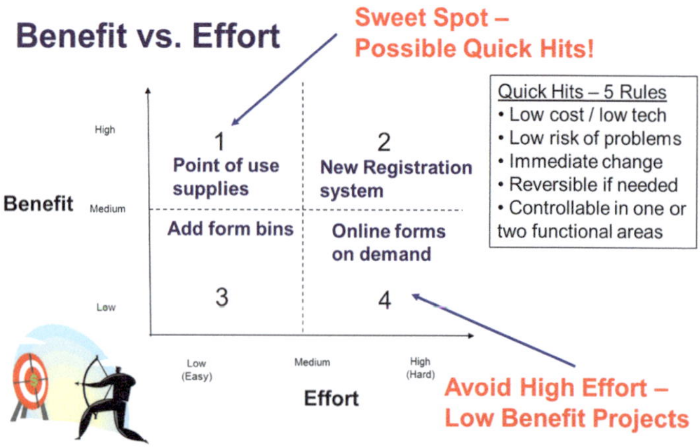

Fig. 6 Benefit effort matrix tool

- Provide standard orders for basic procedures based on chief complaint – eliminate waiting for procedures.
- Install room flags (kanban – see below) to indicate room status – improved communication:

Kanban [2]

A signal to perform a task

- Kanbans take the guesswork out of knowing what to do – visual management.
- Various forms such as bins (empty/full), lights, and outlines around the item "home" location (shadow box).

In the case of the room flag, one of the three flags is pivoted out from the wall. A green flag means the room is ready, a yellow flag means the room needs to be readied for the next patient, and a red flag means the patient is in the room.

Fishbone Diagram

A tool to determine variation and defect root causes (Fig. 7).

The next day, Howard facilitated the use of this tool with the team. It was depicted as follows:

When the map was completed, six items were believed to have the largest impact on throughput. These were circled on

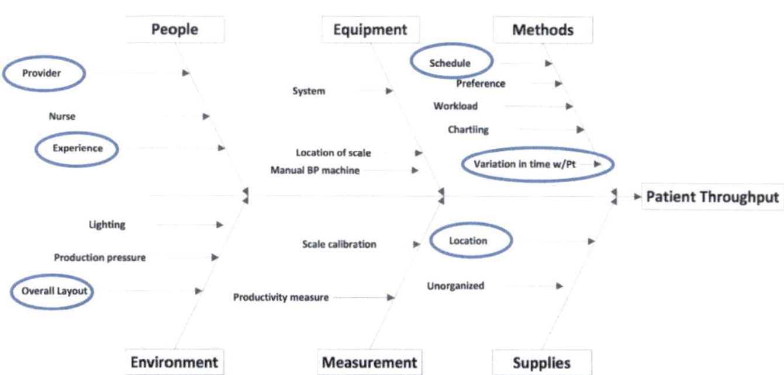

FIG. 7 Clinic fishbone diagram

the diagram. The layout and location of supplies already had targeted interventions so the rest are needed to be investigated to determine if each had significant impact on throughput (lead time).

Six Sigma Tools

Application of statistics to eliminate defects and reduce process variability.

Since the mean is easily understood, it is often the measure used in goal statements; however, it tells us nothing about the variation of the process. The median (middle value of the values when sorted from high to low) is less sensitive to outliers, and in our case, it is 110 min. The reason for the disparity was due to outliers (values farthest from the mean), most notably on the longer visit side. By plotting the distribution, we can "see" the variation and can also obtain a measure of this spread called standard deviation. This is basically the average distance of our points from our mean. In our case, it is 24 min. If we can reduce the standard deviation, we will have less variability in our process, and our patients and staff will have a more predictable experience. We will later look for these sources and put in countermeasures for the ones that affect the process the most.

Statistics can be calculated by hand, but statistical software offers the benefit of providing pictures along with needed statistical information. You can "see" the variation in the following graph (Fig. 8).

Process Capability

Explains how well is our process performing to the "voice of the customer," i.e., customer expectations.

The capability can be expressed as a sigma level that equates to a defect level expressed as DPMO (defects per million opportunities). A Six Sigma process only generates 3.4 defects out of one million times. For most audiences, the use of percentages is the preferred way to explain capability (Table 1).

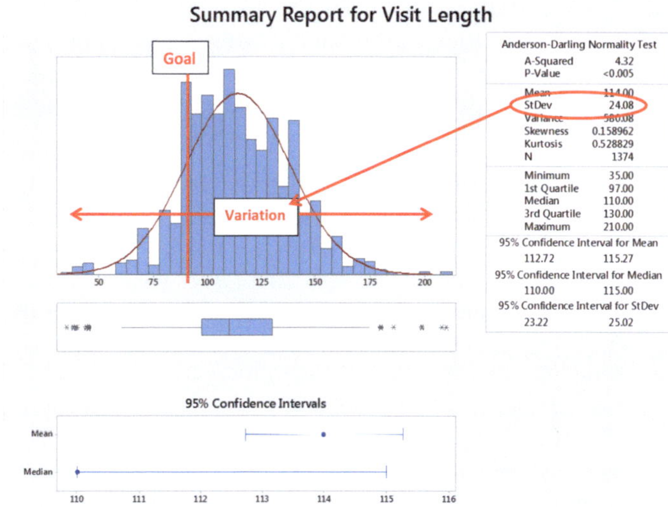

FIG. 8 Graphical summary depicting variation using Minitab

Table 1 Methods to express process capability indices

DPMO	% Defects	Process sigma
691,462	69.1 %	1
308,537	30.8 %	2
66,807	6.7 %	3
6210	0.62 %	4
233	0.02 %	5
3.4	<0.001 %	6

A histogram with customer specification limits is a helpful way of "seeing" the capability of our process. All items outside the lower and upper specification levels are defects. This percentage of data outside of our limits (only an upper limit in this case) was approximately 87 % or less than one sigma. As the graph shows, the mean needs to be centered between the limits and the spread, or variation also needs to be reduced in order to have the data fit between the limits.

The team believed that the various physicians varied in their times spent with patients. Objective data is needed to either reject or fail to reject this hypothesis (Fig. 9):

Hypothesis testing – Statistical tests that determine the probability that a hypothesis is correct.

P value – The probability that the results seen are by chance and chance alone. Smaller P values provide higher confidence that the null hypothesis can be rejected. The P-calculated value is compared to the significance level (or risk we are willing to accept of being incorrect), and if the P value is lower, the null can be rejected and go with the hypothesis.

Which hypothesis test do you use? There are many hypothesis tests to choose from. There are many good statistical references available to help guide you if you

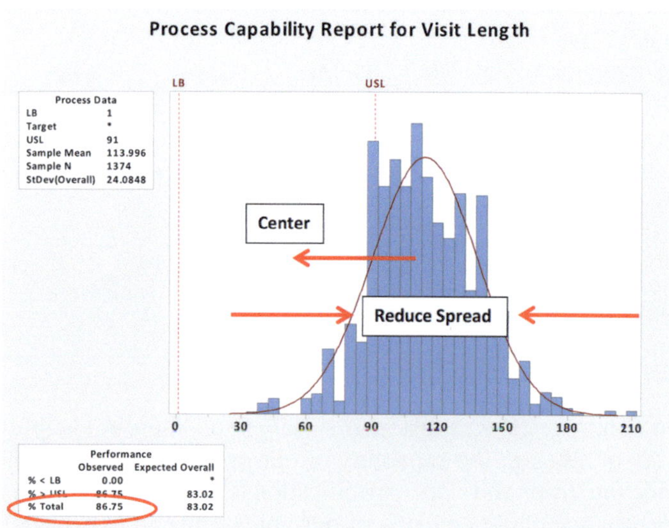

FIG. 9 Minitab® graph depicts the need to reduce both mean and variation

are uncertain of which to use. Factors such as the type of distribution (e.g., normal, lognormal, etc.), analysis in question (centering or spread), and the type of data being investigated are critical in choosing the correct test (Fig. 10).

Various data factors such as the experience of the provider, patients scheduled by time of day, and length of visit by the provider may be analyzed to determine which (if any) have significant impact on the process.

Getting back to our example, if our hypothesis is that there is a statistical difference in the mean lead time between providers, the tool of choice would be ANOVA as the response data type of lead time is a variable data and the six providers (or things we are testing against) represent attribute data.

The analysis is as follows: See Fig. 11.

This graph shows:

- Provider B's visit length is shorter than the others (dots).
- The width of the bars indicates the confidence interval (95 % range of values if additional information was collected).
- Since the P value was less than .05 (significance level), we can reject the null (assumes no differences between provid-

X – Input Factor Data Type	Y - Response Data Type: Variable	Y - Response Data Type: Attribute
Variable	• Correlation • Regression	• Logistic Regression
Attribute	• t-Tests • F-Test • ANOVA	• Chi-Square

FIG. 10 Table for basis hypothesis test selection

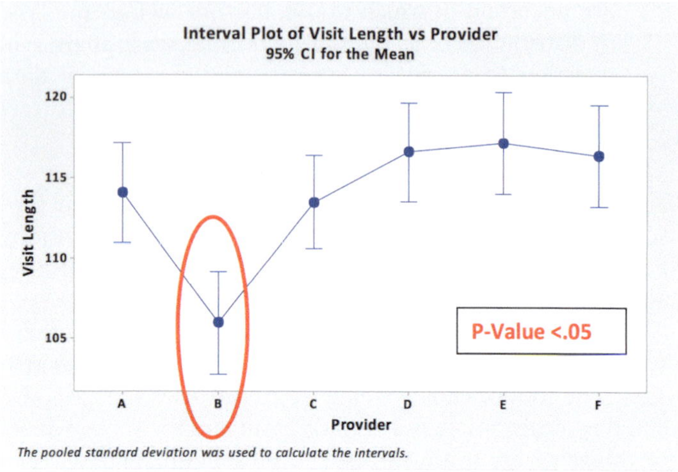

FIG. 11 Minitab® graph of patient visit length by the provider

ers) and conclude that there is a statistical difference between provider B and the others.

Howard presented this to the team and asked, "What makes provider B different from the rest?" This provider had more experience than some but less than the others. Similar statistical analysis indicated the patient mix by complaint and schedule was similar to the others. Howard then told the team the identity of Dr. B. The team suspected it was Bonnie as she appeared to be the most efficient. The team decided to review Bonnie's methods to determine if she had the best practice. Howard, Kate, and the team began to walk step-by-step through Bonnie's approach and shortly thereafter had their answer:

- Upon patient arrival – while they were waiting – only Bonnie had them complete a brief patient visit form that she had created asking specific questions such as:
  - Reason for visit
  - Specific symptoms
  - Length of time they were symptomatic
  - Medications they were taking

- For each of Bonnie's patients, the nurse obtained this list and:
  - Anticipated supplies/equipment related to the visit if not already in the room
  - Informational handout materials that may be needed
- Bonnie reviewed the list prior to entering the room and seeing the patient.

Bonnie said, "I guess I never thought much about it but it helps me focus on the patient." Bonnie's nurse shook her head in agreement. "Best practices like these don't always get shared because there is no time to think about it, let alone discuss it," said Howard. The power of this process is that we use a systemized approach to obtain and analyze data enabling the team to quickly focus on specific problems and arrive at consensus-based solutions.

Improve (DMAIC) or Do (PDCA) Phase

Piloting Interventions

A rapid test of change to learn, adjust as necessary, and retry the agreed-upon changes:

- Piloting on a small scale is beneficial to a complete "roll out" – a safer, more controlled setting.
- Prior to piloting, ensure that all stakeholders are informed in order to minimize confusion or resistance.
- The proper mentality is 20 % think, 40 % do, and 40 % redo – in form, it will most likely not be perfect the first time it is tried.
- Provide an appropriate amount of time for the pilot and meet often to check in and adjust as required.

The team agreed to stay late and establish each intervention listed earlier as well as physician B's best practice. They would then pilot them beginning the next day with a lunch meeting to assess how well they were working or if any modifications were required.

Improve (DMAIC) or Check (PDCA) Phase

The next day at noon, the team briefly met and determined that the only modification needed was to partition off the scale area in the registration room as patient's were self-conscious of staff being in the room while they were being weighed. The decision was made to temporarily relocate the scale to a more secluded area until a suitable partition could be found. Everything else was working well so the pilot continued on those items.

Post-baseline Data

Additional data collected to assess if interventions are yielding the desired benefit.

The team agreed to begin collecting lead time/variation data for the remainder of the day, and the next to determine if the interventions were working. A process capability chart was rerun with the postintervention data to determine if the capability improved (Fig. 12). Note that the capability has improved from 87 % defects at baseline (see earlier chart) vs. 36 % postintervention. Process variation decreased from a standard deviation of 24 at baseline vs. 22 postintervention which is indicative of a more predictable process.

The postintervention ANOVA analysis shows that the differences among providers are no longer statistically different as the P value is now >0.05. In addition, the means of every provider have decreased (Fig. 13).

Box Plot

A graph that depicts centering and the spread of the data by showing quartiles and outliers (Fig. 14).

This graph is helpful in order to "see" the change. The baseline mean of 114 min was far higher than the

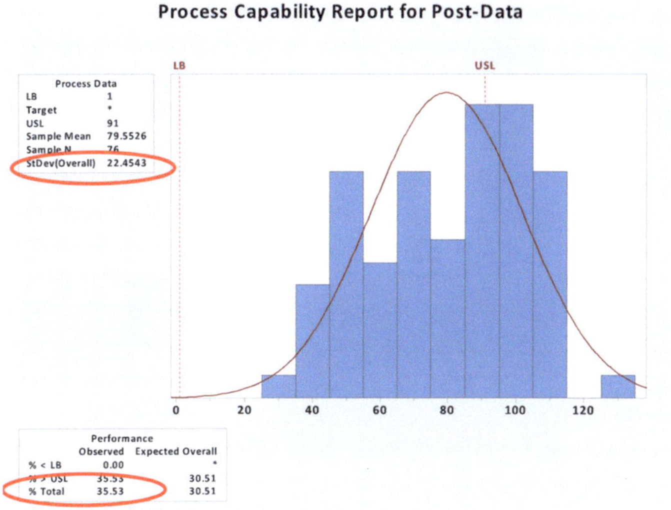

FIG. 12 Minitab® process capability for postintervention data

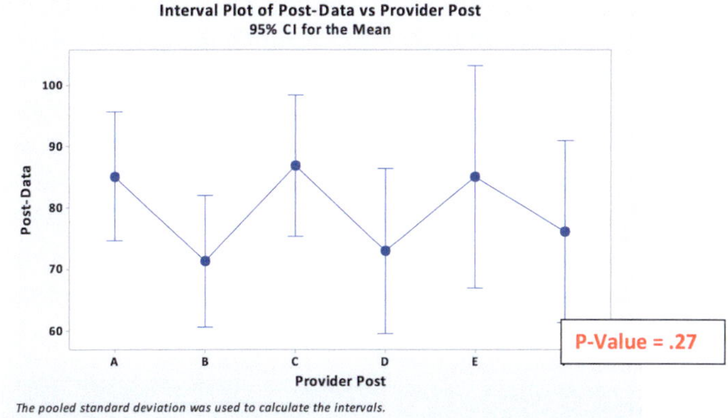

FIG. 13 Minitab® postintervention ANOVA for visit length by the provider

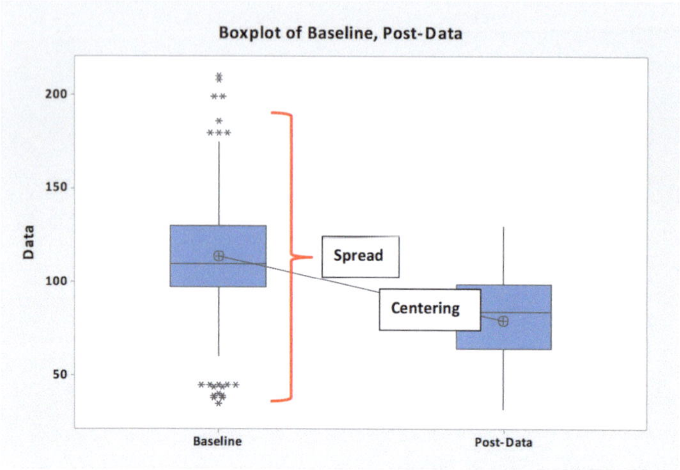

FIG. 14 Minitab® box plot comparing baseline versus postintervention visit length

postintervention time of 80 min. Can we conclude that we have met our goal? More data will be required to be collected in order to declare victory. We will need to measure several weeks of data to ensure our new interventions have truly improved the process. In some cases, additional adjustments or further interventions need to be initiated.

Control (DMAIC) or Act (PDCA) Phase

In order to move to this final stage, the following must occur to systemize the new process:

1. Policies and procedures must be updated to document the changes made.
2. Ongoing measurements must be established:
   (a) Periodic sampling of the key or process metric to ensure sustainability
3. A control plan to document corrective actions if needed.

Process Metric

A leading operational metric that supports the lagging key metric

One of the key interventions in our example that needs to be maintained is the use of the patient visit form. Compliance of this form use was felt to be critical to the continued success of reduced lead times. It was agreed that the forms would be collected for each day in order to compare the number used vs. the number of total visits. A control chart serves as a valuable tool to help monitor this.

The chart below was created with the first 15 days of data. See Fig. 15.

Control chart interpretation:

- Each point shows the day's proportion of forms completed – note each point must be in time series order.
- The initial compliance was low as providers took time to adopt the form.
- The overall chart indicates compliance improved over time and is leveling off at a high rate of performance.

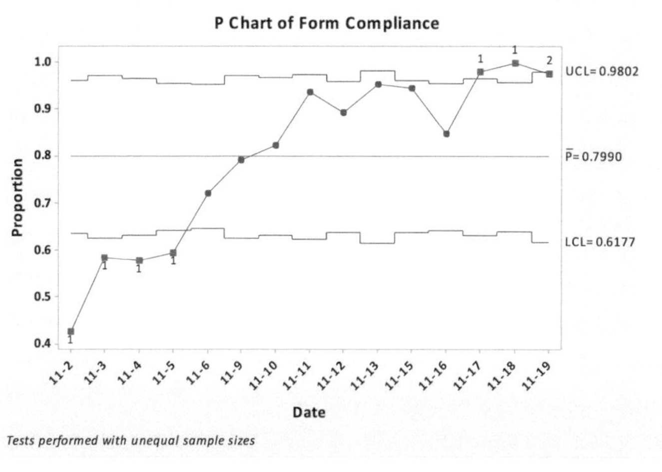

FIG. 15 Minitab® P-chart of patient visit form compliance

Conclusion

Several weeks later, Kate called Howard to tell him that the practice was sustaining shorter lead times ranging between 82 and 92 min. All the hard work had paid off! "This Lean Sigma thing really does work!" said Kate. "Yes it does, the principles may be applied to any process and healthcare is last to the party." "So what are you going to work on next?" asked Howard.

Kaizen [3]

Continuous improvement

Every process must be continually reassessed to ensure that it is meeting and preferably exceeding customer needs and wants. Changing technology and increased customer expectations will continue to steadily "raise the bar." Today's shorter visit lead time will likely be unacceptable in the near future as the competition is improving also. Our charge is to provide a safer healthcare with higher quality, efficiency, and reduced cost. All of these can be continually improved through the use of tools such as Lean Sigma.

If you have any questions about the information covered in this chapter or other medical safety and quality improvement-related topics, please contact us at http://www.medicalqualityandsafetyforum.com. The website will also provide a forum where you can ask specific questions about your safety and medical quality improvement projects or mentor upcoming medical quality leaders.

References

1. Takt – Ohno T. Toyota production system – the length of time it takes to make one piece. Tokyo: Diamond Inc.; 1978.
2. Kanban – Ohno T. Toyota production system – a signal to work – perform a task. Tokyo: Diamond Inc; 1978.
3. Kaizen – Imai M. Kaizen: the key to Japan's competitive success – continuous improvement. New York: McGraw-Hill; 1986.

Part VI
Technical Aspects of Quality Improvement

QI Tools: Epidemiology Basics – Application of Epidemiological Tools to Patient Safety and Quality [1, 2]

Ruchika Goel and Raminder Chadha

Tools

Absolute risk reduction (ARR), Analytical study, ANCOVA, ANOVA, Attributable risk, Available prior literature, Bias, Case–control study, Chi-squared test, Closed population, Cohort study, Confidence interval, Confounding variable, Data collection, Data reporting and monitoring, Descriptive study, Disease frequency measure, Disease natural history, Disease surveillance, Effect modification (interaction), Effectiveness, Epidemiological study, Evidence-based, Experimental study, Hypothesis testing, Incidence rate, Longitudinal analysis, Matching of case and control, Number needed to treat, Observational (nonexperimental) study, Odds ratio (relative odds), *Online Provider Training Module on VTE Prophylaxis*, Open population, Outcome measure, Parametric and non-parametric, Patient safety indicator, Population, Positive and negative predictive values, Power, Predictive modeling, Prevalence, Prospective cohort study, p-values, Quasi-experimental study, Randomized controlled trial

R. Goel (✉)
Division of Pediatric Hematology, The Johns Hopkins Hospital, Baltimore, MD, USA
e-mail: ruchikagoel1@gmail.com

R. Chadha
Johns Hopkins Hospital, Baltimore, MD, USA

L. Atanelov (ed.), *Resident's Handbook of Medical Quality and Safety*, DOI 10.1007/978-3-319-24190-6_31

(RCT), Regression analysis, Risk ratio (relative risk), Risk score, Screening, System-supported, True and false positives, t-test, Types of outcomes, Validity, Variable transformations, Variable types, *VTE Safety Toolkit*

Types of Epidemiological Studies

1. ***Observational (Nonexperimental)***: Observational because there is no individual intervention, treatment, and exposures that occur in a "non-study" environment (i.e., not randomly). Individuals can be observed prospectively, retrospectively, or currently. Observational studies can be designed in two ways:

   Descriptive study design: A type of observational epidemiologic study that has no predetermined hypothesis and simply describes what exists in a population by person, place, or time variables.

   Analytical study design: A type of epidemiologic study which uses comparison groups, which provide baseline data, to quantify the association between exposures and outcomes and test hypotheses about causal relationships:

   (a) Cohort study: Epidemiological study in which subsets of a defined population (cohorts) are identified who are, have been, or in the future may be exposed (or not) to a factor hypothesized to influence the probability of occurrence of any given outcome. Cohort is followed over time, and outcomes ascertained (i.e., disease incidence, death, remission, etc.).

   (b) Case–control study: A type of observational study in which two existing groups differing in outcome (subjects who have a condition/disease (the "cases") and patients who do not have the condition/disease but are otherwise similar (the "controls")) are identified and compared on the basis of some supposed causal attribute.

2. ***Experimental***: Used when epidemiologists have control over the circumstances from the start. For example,

   Randomized controlled trial (RCT): Study where subjects are randomly allocated one or other of the different treatments under study. RCT is often used to test the efficacy or effectiveness of various types of medical intervention and is the gold standard for a clinical trial.

   Quasi-experimental designs: Category of studies that falls between observational and true experimental studies; thus they are called "quasi-experimental studies." In these, there is an intervention, but it is often not completely planned by the person doing the research. Typically, random allocation is not involved.

Types of Populations

Closed Populations

Populations where the members do not change over time.

Open Populations

Most populations change with individuals leaving and others entering; these are referred to as open or dynamic populations.

Measures of Disease Frequency

Incidence Rate

A measure of the frequency with which an event, such as a new case of illness, occurs in a population over a period of time. The denominator is the population at risk; the numerator is the number of new cases occurring during a given time period.

Prevalence

Proportion of population with disease at a specific point in time.

Outcome Measures

Risk Ratio (Relative Risk)

The ratio of the probability of an event occurring in an exposed group to the probability of the event occurring in a comparison, nonexposed group.

$$RR = \frac{p_{\text{event when exposed}}}{p_{\text{event when non-exposed}}}.$$

Odds Ratio (Relative Odds)

The OR represents the odds that an outcome will occur given a particular exposure, compared to the odds of the outcome occurring in the absence of that exposure. Odds ratios are most commonly used in case–control studies; however they can also be used in cross-sectional and cohort study designs as well.

Attributable Risk

Attributable risk is the difference in the rate of a condition between an exposed population and an unexposed population. Attributable risk is mostly calculated in cohort studies, where individuals are assembled on exposure status and followed over a period of time.

Absolute Risk Reduction (ARR)

The change in risk of a given activity or treatment in relation to a control activity or treatment. It is the inverse of the number needed to treat.

Number Needed to Treat

Number of patients needed to be treated for one "cure" = 1/ARR.

Threats to Validity of an Epidemiological Study

Confounding

When a noncausal association is observed between a given exposure and outcome as a result of the influence of a third variable, it is termed confounding, with the third variable termed a confounding variable. A confounding variable is causally associated with the outcome of interest, and non-causally or causally associated with the exposure, but is not an intermediate variable in the causal pathway between exposure and outcome.

Effect Modification (Interaction)

Interaction occurs when the direction or magnitude of an association between two variables differs due to the effect of a third variable. It may reflect a cumulative effect of multiple risk factors, which are not acting independently, and produce a greater or lesser effect than the sum of the effects of each factor acting on its own.

Bias

A statistic is biased if it is calculated in such a way that it is systematically different from the population parameter of interest, e.g., selection bias and nonresponse bias.

The International Journal for Quality in Health Care outlined an "'Epidemiological Risk Factor Model For Analysis Of Patient Safety Outcome" by seeking to uncover statistical associations, at the population level, between putative risk factors and outcomes of interest (Table 1).

TABLE 1 Epidemiological risk factor model for the analysis of patient safety incidents

Core disciplines	Epidemiology
Typical outcome of interest	(i) Health problem
	(ii) Incident/event
Unit of analysis	Population or sample of events
Design of investigation	Case–control study
	Prospective study
	Randomized trial
Assessment of causes	Standardized measurement of risk factors
Attribution of causality	Statistical association between risk factor and outcome
Threats to validity	Bias
	Effect modification
	Confounding
Key advantages	Generalizability
	Capacity to examine joint effects of several risk factors
	Quantification of the strength of risk factors

Case Example of Application of Epidemiological Tools to Improvement of Patient Safety Outcomes

We will use the example of development and use of venous thromboembolism (VTE) as a core patient safety outcome measure to outline an example of applicability of epidemiological tools to improve patient safety outcomes.

Venous thromboembolism (VTE) prevention, diagnosis, and treatment require coordination of care across multiple providers supported by a system that assists in the process of delivering and tracking outcomes of care. The VTE measures were developed as a result of the "National Consensus Standards for the Prevention and Care of Deep Vein Thrombosis (DVT)" project between The Joint Commission and the National Quality Forum (NQF). The measures were tested through a multiphased approach.

As of today, six VTE measures are endorsed by the NQF and are approved as a core measure set for use by The Joint Commission and impact each stage of management including the preventive, diagnostic, and therapeutic algorithms. These measures include VTE Prophylaxis, VTE Intensive Care Unit VTE Prophylaxis, VTE Thromboembolism Patients with Anticoagulation Overlap Therapy, VTE Patients Receiving Unfractionated Heparin with Dosages/Platelet Count, VTE Warfarin Therapy Discharge Instructions, and VTE Hospital-Acquired Potentially Preventable Venous Thromboembolism.

Determinants of Predictors of VTE in Hospitals and Strategies for Prevention and Surveillance: Example of Stepwise Application of Epidemiological Tools

1. Study design, data collection, and analysis of vital records: Using a "case–control study design and 1:2 matching of case and control," cases were selected from the JHU hospitalization data case. We **reviewed available prior literature** to guide the selection of variables that were potential predictors.
2. Disease surveillance: In order to establish patterns of DVT occurrence and recurrence, **disease surveillance with proper data reporting and monitoring** of each new case as a **patient safety indicator** is done.
3. Identification of individuals, subgroups, or populations at risk of developing certain diseases: We used regression analysis for **predictive modeling** for weighted estimates to identify the predictors of VTE in hospitalized setting.
4. Providing data necessary for health planning and decision making: Based on the above analysis, a **risk score** was

developed which is being used for **screening** patients at high risk of VTE development.

5. Intervention: Patients deemed at high risk for VTE development are offered mechanical of pharmacological prophylaxis for VTE. One example of operating this is hospital specific use of the **evidence-based**, **system-supported, interactive** *VTE Safety Toolkit* – which includes diagnostic, preventive, and therapeutic algorithms – and the *Online Provider Training Module on VTE Prophylaxis*, which can be a web-based VTE educational intervention for all providers.
6. Evaluation of effectiveness of existing or newly proposed treatment: A **prospective cohort study** is currently in progress to compare the rates of VTE in populations with and without prophylaxis measures.
7. Evaluation of health programs: Long-term **longitudinal analysis** of clinical characteristics of patients who develop VTE during hospitalizations can help provide information on **natural history of disease** as well as **effectiveness** of various preventative strategies.

Summary

The staggering number of patients harmed by preventable medical errors highlights importance of patient safety. Correct knowledge and applicability of epidemiological tools as outlined above to patient safety/quality can lead to significantly improved patient safety and quality outcomes.

If you have any questions about the information covered in this chapter or other medical safety and quality improvement-related topics, please contact us at http://www.medicalqualityandsafetyforum.com. The website will also provide a forum where you can ask specific questions about your safety and medical quality improvement projects or mentor upcoming medical quality leaders.

Reference

1. Hulley SB, Cummings SR, et al. Designing clinical research. 3rd ed. New York: Lippincott, Williams and Wilkins; 2013.
2. Gordis L. Epidemiology. 4th ed. New York: Saunders Elsevier; 2009.

Introduction to Data Analysis for QI Projects

Marlis Gonzalez-Fernandez

Tools
Data collection, outcome and secondary variable selection, types of variables, dichotomous, discrete, continuous, categorical, numerical, hypothesis testing, measures, ratio, mean, median, percent, proportion, statistically significant, 2x2 table, chi-squared, ANOVA, ANCOVA, Fisher's test, small sample size, p-value, alternative hypothesis, logarithmic transformation, square root transformation, non-parametric statistics, power, sample size, confidence interval, logistical regression, linear regression, false negatives, false positives, positive predictive value, negative predictive value, sensitivity, specificity

The purpose of this chapter is to introduce the reader to basic data analysis principles that can be helpful in exploring data, determining the significance of findings, and deriving conclusions.

Without sound data, any analysis effort will be fraught with challenges. Having a clear question prior to starting data

M. Gonzalez-Fernandez (✉)
Department of Physical Medicine and Rehabilitation, John Hopkins Hospital, Baltimore, MD, USA
e-mail: mgonzal5@jhmi.edu

L. Atanelov (ed.), *Resident's Handbook of Medical Quality and Safety*, DOI 10.1007/978-3-319-24190-6_32

collection allows researchers the opportunity to determine what data needs to be collected, time frames, and feasibility.

Fall Prevention as an Example

If one is interested in reducing falls in medical settings, we need to define operationally what that means. Perhaps we can ask: Can the number of falls in the neurology floor be reduced by 25 % by using the ABC fall prevention protocol?

This question helps us identify the various pieces of information one needs. First, we need to know the kind of data that needs to be collected. In the example above, we are interested in the number of falls. This could be falls per month, number of patient falls by patients admitted, etc. Choosing a particular measure will help determine the time span during which data needs to be collected and information needed to make such a selection. Are falls in the neurology floor frequent enough to allow for reliable fall rate measurement and comparison month to month? What would be the pre- and post-intervention period? What change in rates is clinically meaningful?

It might be useful not only to know the fall rate in the neurology unit but also the personal characteristics, admission diagnosis, or comorbidities of the people that are falling. We know that we are interested in reducing falls, but perhaps there are other related questions such as: Are the people falling older? Are they more likely to have one admission diagnosis versus another? Are they overall sicker (have more comorbidities)?

Data Collection

In the aforementioned example, we are interested in the number of falls and how other personal, admission, or systems of care factors affect fall rates. Falls are discrete events that can easily be counted. Perhaps it is meaningful to express fall as a rate (falls per month, falls per 1000 patient days) or proportion (# of patient falls a year or # of patients admitted a year). Deciding on what measure is most meaningful depends on the circumstances, the frequency of the event or outcome being studied, and available measures or benchmarks, among other factors. Once the, measure to be used is decided the data analysis plan will follow.

Selection of Outcome Variables and Secondary Variables

If we assume that a decision was made to use the fall rate per 1000 patient days to track falls (as data is often reported in the literature using this measure), a data analysis plan can be devised. Perhaps the main comparison of interest is between the falls 6 months prior to the intervention versus 6 months after the fall prevention intervention was established.

It is important to determine other factors that are likely to influence the fall rate and that are not or cannot be addressed by the intervention. For example, one third of adults age 65 or older fall each year [1]. Consequently, if the neurology unit admits a large proportion of patients 65 years of age or older, the results of the intervention may appear discouraging, unless the rates are calculated separately for people younger than 65 years of age and 65 years of age or older. Other factors that may affect the rates and obscure findings should be considered based on clinical expertise and the best available evidence. Examples of possible variables that may be collected in a fall prevention study are detailed in Table 1.

Data Summary and Analysis

Descriptive statistics are used to provide a basic summary of the data being studied. If we continue following the example above, data should have been collected on several key vari-

TABLE 1 Examples of variables in a fall prevention study

Variable	Measure (examples)
Falls	Present/absent
Number of patients admitted to the floor every day	Count of patients in admission census (checked at the same time every day)
Nursing hours	Hours worked by nurses each day (total)
Hospital length of stay (for each patient)	Days (including partial days)
Age	Years
Admitting diagnosis	Each diagnosis perhaps categorized as affecting mobility or cognition
Comorbidity measure	Diagnosis count, Charlson Index, AHRQ Comorbidity index
Presence of delirium/ dementia	Yes/no

ables or factors related to in-hospital falls. The variables detailed in Table 1 need to be summarized to compare before and after the intervention (Table 2). The measures or statistics used to summarize the data are based on the data type to which each variable belongs. For some variables, it might be necessary to create categories as suggested for age above.

Hypothesis Testing

Once the data is summarized and categorized, differences between groups can emerge. Once the fall rate prior to and after the intervention is calculated, we need to determine if there are differences and if such differences are significant (statistically) and clinically meaningful.

Let's assume that at first glance there is a difference in the rates that would be considered clinically important. Is that difference statistically significant? Can that difference be explained by other factors besides the intervention?

TABLE 2 Examples of descriptive statistics for the sample variables

Variable	Data type	Statistic
Falls (count)	Dichotomous	Falls/patient days (ratio), proportion or percentage of patients falling per unit time (month, year, etc.)
Number of patients admitted to the floor every day	Discrete	Patients/24 h (measured at 12:00 midnight)
Nursing hours	Continuous	Hours/patient (ratio)
Hospital length of stay (for each patient)	Continuous	Median or ME admission days, mean admission days
Age	Continuous[a]	Median or mean age
Admitting diagnosis	Categorical	Percent of patients with a high-risk fall diagnosis
Comorbidity measure	Numerical (index or count)	Mean or median number of diagnoses, mean or median of comorbidity index
Presence of delirium/ dementia	Dichotomous	Proportion or percentage of all patients with the diagnosis

[a]May be separated into categories. For example, <65 years of age or ≥65 years of age. Then the proportion or percentage of patients in each category can be presented

To determine if the rates are statistically different before and after the intervention, a statistical test can be applied. In the current example, the variable of interest can only be one of two options; it was either present or absent. Thus, a classic 2×2 table can be generated (Table 3).

The statistical test applied to the data available from Table 3 depends on the count in each cell (gray area). Chi-squared statistics (or 2 sample tests of proportions) would be the test applicable to these data. One consideration is sample size. If the events are infrequent or the sample size is small

Table 3 Table format for falls analysis

		Falls		
		Present	**Absent**	**Total**
Time point	Before intervention	a	b	
	Post-intervention	c	d	
	Total			

(any cell in Table 3 with <5), a Fisher's exact test should be used. For comparisons between two groups of numerical data (discrete or continuous data such as age or fasting blood sugar level), t-tests can be used (assuming that the data is normally distributed). If more than three groups are being compared, one-way analysis of variance (ANOVA) may be appropriate. Categorical variables with more than two categories (such as race or blood type) can also be analyzed using chi-squared statistics.

The results of these tests are p-values. The p-value represents the probability of obtaining the observed results when the null hypothesis (usually stating that there is no difference) is true. In this case, it would be the probability that there is no difference in falls before and after the intervention. The smaller the p-value, the greater the probability that the alternative hypothesis (in this case, that the intervention resulted in fall reduction) is true. By convention, a p-value of 0.05 or smaller is considered statistically significant and would result in rejecting the null hypothesis. Depending on the data being analyzed, the 0.05 p-value can be considered too large and may be set instead at 0.01 or 0.001. This is particularly important when analyzing very large data sets.

Generally speaking, classical tests of hypotheses are based on several assumptions. When using any of the statistical tools mentioned in this chapter, we suggest that the details that relate to the test are studied to insure that the test can be used based on the characteristics of the data. One of the most common assumptions is that the data is normally distributed. In cases where this assumption is not true, nonparametric statistics should be used. Another alternative is mathematically transforming the data to meet the assumption prior to using the statistical test. Common examples of transformations include logarithmic or square root transformations. Please see the references at the end of this chapter for more details.

It is important to mention that there are other factors to consider when deciding the significance of a particular set of data. One such factor is statistical power. Using our example, power would answer the question: How likely are we to statistically *reject* the hypothesis that the intervention reduces falls when in fact it does? Power is largely affected by the sample size and the effect size one is trying to measure. Thus, it is important to consider power early in the study to determine the appropriate sample size. The nuances of power calculation are beyond the scope of this chapter. Multiple power and sample size calculators are **available online, e.g.,** http://www.stat.ubc.ca/~rollin/stats/ssize/ **or** http://www.sealedenvelope.com/power.

Also, please note that the confidence interval of the results have to be considered. There is a difference between a 95 % confidence interval (CI) being 3.14 to $\pm$0.02 vs. 3.14 $\pm$ 2.14. In the former case, we are pretty confident (95 % chance) that the calculated value is well approximated by the calculation to the first decimal place with narrow confidence interval, so the calculated value is pretty close to a real value, whereas in the latter case, we can say that we are 95 % confident that the real value is somewhere between 1.00 and 5.28 (wide confidence interval), i.e., the calculated value is a very rough approximation of the real value.

Other Statistical Tools

In the case of falls, we are interested in the effect multiple factors have on falls; in this case, basic tests of the hypothesis do not provide a full picture. If we chose to collect data on every patient admitted over a period of time and whether that patient fell during an admission or not (a yes/no categorical variable), a logistic regression may be used. A logistic regression would allow the effect that multiple factors may have, as a whole, on the outcome of interest. As we stated above, factors affecting falls may include the number of patients admitted to a floor every day, nursing hours, hospital length of stay, age, admitting diagnosis, medical comorbidities, or the presence of delirium/dementia. These factors are important in that the effect of the intervention may be obscured. For example, if the patients admitted after the intervention was implemented are overall older than the patients that were admitted in the hospital prior to the intervention, we might see that the intervention had no effect (or even that there were more falls after the intervention!). Using a tool like logistic regression, we can determine if a particular factor increased the odds of someone falling or decreased them. The mathematical underpinnings of this test are beyond the scope of this chapter. In the most basic terms, we are using a series of factors to determine the odds of the outcome of interest happening (in this case, falls) based on those factors. The results of a logistic regression provide us the odds of the outcome occurring if the factor is present compared to the odds of the outcome if the factor is absent (odds ratio) and lets us know if that effect is statistically significant.

In some instances, the variable of interest is not categorical. Perhaps we are interested in the effect an intervention has on the reduction of fasting blood sugar levels. In this case, a logistic regression would not be appropriate. A linear regression is one of the most commonly used tools to study the effect multiple variables have on a continuous outcome variable. Care should be placed on the assumptions that this type of analysis is to insure appropriate use.

Another tool that can be used to determine the effect of a factor on the relationship between a continuous or numerical outcome variable and a categorical variable is analysis of covariance (ANCOVA). This analysis would be appropriate, for example, when one is interested in fasting blood sugar by categorical groups (perhaps people on a diabetic diet vs. those who are not) and when another factor may be of influence. In this example, if the population being studied was patients with rheumatoid arthritis, the use of corticosteroids would have a great influence on fasting blood sugar and has to be considered.

Test Characteristics

Identifying patients that are likely to have a particular outcome based on a set of known parameters may be important in the context of quality improvement. Continuing with our original example, we would like to know how accurate is the combination of factors in predicting what patients are likely to fall. Perhaps if we are able to correctly identify the patients that are going to fall, we can concentrate our prevention efforts on those people. The factors of interest in this case are analog to a test and have to be compared against the truth (whether the patient really falls or not). Table 4 can help us demonstrate some of the analysis that may be used.

We would like to know how likely this "test" is to correctly identify the people that fell from all the people that fell, the true positive rate, or sensitivity. Conversely, we are also interested in how many patients that do not fall are correctly identified, the

TABLE 4 Data required for test characteristic calculation

		True falls			
		Yes	No	Total	
Falls test	Positive	a	b	a + b	PPV = a/a + b
	Negative	c	d	c + d	NPV = d/c + d
	Total	a + c	b + d		
		Sensitivity= a/a + c	Specificity= d/b + d		

true negative rate, or specificity. A good test will maximize both sensitivity and specificity resulting in very few false negatives (c) and false positives (b). It may also be useful to know the proportion of all the people who test positive who actually fall, that is, the positive predictive value (PPV), and the proportion of people who test negative who actually will not fall, that is, the negative predictive value (NPV). The basic calculations needed to obtain these values are detailed in Table 4.

Conclusion

Statistical tests are powerful tools to use to detect differences when implementing quality improvement efforts. The information included in this chapter is introductory and intended to be used as a guide when deciding what data to collect and what information will be useful to have when the project is completed. All complex projects should recruit the assistance of statisticians who can understand the available data and its limitations in the context of the statistics to be used. For those interested in more details on the tests and techniques mentioned above, please refer to the suggested reading list below.

Other Resources

Rosner B. Fundamentals of biostatistics. 7th ed. Boston: Brooks/Cole; 2010.

Dawson B, Trapp RG. Basic & clinical biostatistics. 4th ed. New York: Lange Medical Books-McGraw-Hill; 2004.

Motulsky H. Intuitive biostatistics: a non-mathematical guide to statistical thinking. 3rd ed. New York: Oxford University Press; 2014.

Daniel WW, Cross CL. Biostatistics: a foundation for analysis in the Health Sciences. 10th ed. Indianapolis: Wiley; 2013.

Summary Table: Data Types and Common Statistical Tests

Data type	Subcategories	Example	Numeric values	Hypothesis testing	Multiple variable analysis	Examples of data display
Nominal	Dichotomous (binary)	Yes/no Present/absent	0, 1[a]	Chi-squared	Risk ratios Logistic regression	Contingency tables Bar charts
	Categorical	Racial/ethnic background, blood type	0, 1, 2, etc.[a] One unique numeric identifier per category	Chi-squared	Multinomial regression	Proportion or percentage tables
Ordinal		Likert scales[b], severity of disease scales	0, 1, 2, etc.[c]		Spearman rank correlation or ordinal regression	Proportion or percentage tables
Numerical	Discrete	Number of births or events	Integers		Poisson regression	Stem and leaf plots Frequency tables Histograms Boxplots
	Continuous	Age Hemoglobin	Real numbers	T-tests	Correlation coefficient Linear regression	

[a]By convention, numeric label is arbitrary
[b]For example, strongly agree, agree, neutral, disagree, strongly disagree
[c]Numbers are arbitrary but ranking or order matters

If you have any questions about the information covered in this chapter or other medical safety and quality improvement-related topics, please contact us at http://www.medicalqualityandsafetyforum.com. The website will also provide a forum where you can ask specific questions about your safety and medical quality improvement projects or mentor upcoming medical quality leaders.

References

1. Tromp AM, Pluijm SMF, Smit JH, et al. Fall-risk screening test: a prospective study on predictors for falls in community-dwelling elderly. J Clin Epidemiol. 2001;54(8):837–44.

Survey Methodology

Phillip H. Phan

Tools
R statistical language, data loading, variable types, loops, continuous data, power analysis, descriptive statistics, t-test, non-parametrics, ANOVA, ANCOVA, regressions, correlations, non-continuous data, chi-squared test, frequencies, cross-tables, data writing, sig sigma functions in R
Online References for R
LISREL
Qualtrics™
SurveyMonkey™

Introduction

Surveys are a cornerstone technique in healthcare services research methods. Often, it is difficult to make a theoretical and/or empirical case for a direct causal relationship between

P.H. Phan (✉)
Carey Business School, John Hopkins Hospital,
100 International Drive, Baltimore, MD 21202, USA
e-mail: pphan@jhu.edu

L. Atanelov (ed.), *Resident's Handbook of Medical Quality and Safety*, DOI 10.1007/978-3-319-24190-6_33

improvements in organizational processes or individual behaviors and clinical outcomes. Clinical outcomes are multidimensional and multifactorial. Although randomized control group designs can partially solve this problem, the combination of patients' genotypic and phenotypic characteristics makes disease progression, and therefore clinical outcomes, difficult to compare across patients. Additionally, the heterogeneity in case mix in a typical hospital ward, intensive care unit, or emergency department across time can make the link between organizational improvements and clinical outcomes indirect at best. Typically, the indirect causal relationships are mediated by changes in individual (e.g., test-ordering decisions) and organizational (e.g., teaming) behavior. Surveys are employed to measure the direct outcomes of organizational improvement interventions. This technique allows the researcher to measure psychometrically valid responses at the individual, team, and unit level to changes in organizational policies, procedures, and structures.

This guide assumes that the researcher has already established a theory of action, with hypotheses, for why the intervention or observed changes in organizational design or process are expected to influence the decisions and/or behaviors of the survey population. It is critical to note that without a clear theory of action, it is not possible to design a survey that will yield meaningful data [1].

The most common form of surveys is the written questionnaire survey. This is easily deployed through online platforms such as SurveyMonkey™ or Qualtrics™ or paper and pencil forms. Unless the phenomenon under study is very complex, the written questionnaire survey is preferred. Face-to-face, telephone, and observational surveys are also used in healthcare services research, but these tend to be time intensive and subject to observer bias and often do not allow the researcher to collect enough data to establish statistical sampling robustness.

The construction of a theoretically valid and empirically reliable written questionnaire survey follows four well-established steps [2]. First, the researcher must create an item pool to measure the constructs of interest. Next, the researcher must design the survey instrument. Then, the researcher must deploy the instrument and collect the data for analysis. Finally, the researcher must establish the reliability and construct validity of the data collected.

Creating an Item Pool

The item pool (i.e., the questions) comprising a survey can be created through a variety of channels. A common mistake that researchers make is to simply adopt a previously constructed survey without regard to the similarity of the prior target population with the current target population or research question(s) the prior survey was originally designed to answer. Therefore, the first step in constructing the item pool is to conduct a thorough literature review of previous studies. Attention should be paid to context, survey population, and time frame in those studies. Given that healthcare organizations are unique (due to specific institutional arrangements between providers and payers, government regulation at the local level, and population demographics served by the institution), researchers must be careful when adopting previously used surveys. Another way to create an item pool is to interview a subset of the target population, the client(s) for which the survey is being conducted, and/or other experts in the research question.

Designing the Survey Instrument

Once the item pool is created, the following should be noted in designing the questions and structure of the survey [3]:

1. Each construct must be measured with multiple items that are anticipated to tap the same psychological dimension. For example, if one is attempting to measure *resistance to change*, several affirmative and negative questions should be posed to the respondents. These items should converge around the same construct in the post-survey factor analysis.

2. There is a tension between the length of survey, sample size, and stability of the measures. The more items in the survey, the more likely that the measures will be stable across respondents. However, the more items in the survey, the less enthusiastic the respondents in filling in the form. Finally, the more items, the larger the required sample size to achieve a reasonable power of the test. The rule of thumb is 10x the number of respondents for each item, so that a ten-item questionnaire would require at least 100 respondents. The implication of this statistical constraint is that good survey questionnaires should be tightly focused on a specific research question to be useful.
3. Avoid double-barreled questions. That is, each question should only ask for one piece of information.
4. Avoid stating questions in double negatives or double positives.
5. Use a Likert scale (five-point response scale) and ensure the anchor descriptors of agreement or disagreement are symmetrical on both ends of the scale [4]. A key assumption for Likert scales is that the responses on the scale are equidistant in valence to each other.
6. Researchers sometimes use a cumulative Guttman scale (seven-point response scale) in which agreement with a particular response on the scale indicates agreement with the responses prior to or after that particular response on the same scale. If one uses such a scale, understand that each response represents a cumulative (dis)agreement to the lower (higher)-level responses on the scale; therefore, be careful.
7. Do not use category headings to organize the questionnaire. Category or section headings can bias the responses. Instead, all the items in the questionnaire should be presented together so that respondents will not be able to guess the hypotheses.
8. Avoid language that can generate social desirability biases. Social desirability occurs when a respondent feels that responding a certain way will generate a negative impression of his social image. For example, a question such as "I

care a lot about patient safety" is bound to generate a "strongly agree" response from the survey population. Additionally, one can anticipate very little variance in that response. The reason is that to disagree would cast the respondent in an unfavorable light and therefore be perceived as "socially undesirable."

9. Try to anticipate if one could reasonably expect a wide range of responses to a question. If one does not think that the target population will produce a wide range of responses to a question, don't use the question (it would be a waste of statistical degrees of freedom).
10. Include manipulation checks in the survey instrument. For example, to see if respondents are paying attention to the text in the question, the researcher can word the question in such a way that the responses are reverse coded (i.e., reverse the anchor points on the scale for some questions). The use of repetitive questions, worded in different ways, is sometimes used to check for inconsistent responses. Build such checks into the questionnaire, so that one can analyze the data later on for consistency in response.
11. Always pilot test the questionnaire with a small group from the target population. One can formally pilot test the questionnaire by deploying it and then analyzing the resulting data for distribution and other **sample** statistics. The advantage of doing this is that one can obtain data about the mean/variance characteristics of the dependent variable that will allow one to calculate the optimal sample size of the survey population [5, 6]. The survey can also be informally pilot tested by conducting a focus group with a small group of respondents. This technique allows one to detect poorly designed questions.

Deploying the Survey Instrument

Deploying the survey instrument requires proper planning. There must be consideration of the timing, insight into the propensity of the target population to respond, and data collection protocols.

Typically, weekends and holidays are bad times for a survey to be deployed. In an academic center, major events in the calendar such as interviewing season (for residency programs), graduation, and the end-of-year period are also bad times for deploying a survey if one needed a high response rate. There are a number of techniques to increase response rate such as requesting permission from the survey population to solicit responses, sending reminders 1 week and 3 weeks after initial deployment of the survey, deploying the written survey in focus groups or face-to-face meetings, and incentives such as random drawings for prizes. We know that anonymous surveys tend to report higher responses than non-anonymous surveys. However, if the data of a survey is to be used with other data (such as electronic health records), identity of the respondent may be necessary. In this case, assurances of confidentiality and anonymity in reporting (through post-data collection de-identification) need to be stated in the explanatory paragraph of the instrument. Generally speaking, these measures would have been included in the Institutional Review Board application for authorization to conduct the research.

Whether the target population will respond fully to the questionnaire is a function of how the questionnaire is designed and whether the research question will appeal to the interests of the respondents [7]. Pilot testing is very important for this reason. It will ensure that the questionnaire is positioned in the most favorable light and that the interests of the respondents in completing the questionnaire are anticipated. Oftentimes, prior to the creation of the survey instrument, researchers may spend time in the "field" to observe the phenomenon in situ. This may include shadowing practitioners, **process** mapping, attending morbidity and mortality conferences, attending planning meetings, speaking with patients or patient families, and so on. By doing this, the researcher will also benefit from using the right language and terms of art when writing the questions for the survey. Another benefit to the researcher is to familiarize her with the culture and demographics of the target population so that the insights into their concerns and interests can better inform the design of the questionnaire.

Consideration of how the data will be collected should occur *before* the survey is deployed. The easiest method for data collection and curation is through an online survey platform such as Qualtrics™ or SurveyMonkey™. These applications allow the researcher to design surveys that move a respondent logically through the questionnaire while providing basic error trapping. They allow the researcher to track responses and to include manipulation checks (i.e., questions to detect random responses, inconsistent responses, and the like). The trade-off with using online survey tools is the high incidence of incomplete responses and potential technical failures (lost Internet connections, incompatible browsers, etc.) that can introduce bias and noise into the data. Additionally, if an instrument is complex, paper and pencil forms have been shown to be more reliable, especially if the survey is completed in the presence of the researcher that can answer clarification questions. When using a paper and pencil form, the researcher must plan for how the forms should be conveyed, and confidentiality is protected in the chain of custody.

Establishing Measurement Reliability and Validity

Once the survey instrument has been pilot tested and deployed and the responses collected, the following steps must be followed to establish the reliability of the responses and the validity of the measures [8].

To establish reliability of the questions, the first step is to use exploratory factor analysis (EFA) to examine the data structure. Factor analysis allows the researcher to determine if the items that are meant to measure a particular construct "hang together" in a meaningful way. The factor analysis should show that the items belonging to the same construct will load together in the factor matrix while those that do not belong will not load together.

The next step is to conduct a reliability analysis using Cronbach's alpha [9] to examine the stability of the items for each measure. For an established scale (e.g., if one adapted a well-known scale from previous studies, such as the introversion/extroversion scale), the desired alpha should be better than .70. For a new scale developed for the study, an alpha of better than .60 is acceptable. If multiple respondents are used to measure a unit-level response, the researcher should also calculate a reliability ρ (rho) quotient to establish the consistency of the responses across informants.

The final step is to establish construct validity using confirmatory factor analysis (CFA). A popular statistical package to use for CFA is LISREL. LISREL is used to extract the factors (or constructs) embedded in a dataset and to calculate the coefficient of correlation between the factors. Those factors that are supposed to be distinct constructs should report statistically insignificant and near zero correlations (discriminant validity), while those factors that are supposed to measure related constructs should report statistically significant and meaningful correlations (convergent validity). Additionally, the LISREL procedure should produce factors that comprise items that should "hang together" as expected in the theory.

Summary

The use of survey questionnaires is a common technique for data collection in health services research. Survey design, deployment, and testing follow a well-defined four-step process. This includes creating the item pool, designing the questionnaire, deploying the questionnaire and collecting the data, and verifying the data reliability and theoretical validity of the measures in the instrument. The design of the instrument should be completed prior to the introduction of any intervention (rather than as an afterthought). Generally speaking, to show evidence of impact, the researcher must deploy a pre-intervention and post-intervention version of the survey, preferably with a control (nonintervention group). Therefore, the design of an intervention, while clinically important (and even urgent), needs to take place in parallel with the design of the data collection protocol if evidence of impact needs to be established.

If you have any questions about the information covered in this chapter or other medical safety and quality improvement-related topics, please contact us at http://www.medicalqualityandsafetyforum.com. The website will also provide a forum where you can ask specific questions about your safety and medical quality improvement projects or mentor upcoming medical quality leaders.

References

1. Zeller RA, Carmines EG. Measurement in the social sciences: the link between theory and data. Cambridge, UK: Cambridge University Press; 1980.
2. Dillman DA, Smyth JD, Christian LM. Internet, phone, mail, and mixed-mode surveys: the tailored design method. 4th ed. New York: Wiley; 2014.
3. Fowler F. Improving survey questions: design and evaluation, Applied social research methods series, vol. 38. Thousand Oaks: Sage; 1995.
4. van Alphen A, Halfens R, Hasman A, Imbos T. Likert or Rasch? Nothing is more applicable than good theory. J Adv Nurs. 1994;20:196–201.
5. Walter SD, Eliasziw M, Donner A. Sample size and optimal designs for reliability studies. Stat Med. 1998;17(1):101–10.
6. Cohen J. Statistical power analysis for the behavioral sciences. 2nd ed. New York: Routledge; 2013.
7. Hambleton RK, Swaminathan H, Rogers HJ. Fundamentals of item response theory. Newbury Park: Sage; 1991.

8. Carmines EG, Zeller RA. Reliability and validity assessment, Sage University paper series on quantitative applications in the social sciences, vol. 07–17. Newbury Park: Sage; 1979.
9. Cronbach LJ. Coefficient alpha and the internal structure of tests. Psychometrika. 1951;16:297–333.

Using R for Statistics: A Beginner's Manual

Andre Cassell

> **Tools**
>
> Installing R, load data into R, R interface/console, commands, expressions, data frame, objects, vectors, lists, operator, "for" loop, continuous data, discrete data, analyzing data, power analysis, descriptive statistics, visualization, comparison of two groups, t test, nonparametrics, p-value, Mann-Whitney U test, Wilcoxon Rank Sum Test, Kruskal-Wallis test, ANOVA, ANCOVA, Correlations, linear regression, non-continuous data, Fisher test, Chi-Square test, frequencies, cross tables, Poison regression, Spearman rank correlation, how to write a file, six sigma functions in R.

A. Cassell (✉)
Department of Physical Medicine and Rehabilitation,
John Hopkins Hospital,
600 North Wolfe Street, Suite 160, Baltimore, MD 21287, USA
e-mail: acassel5@jhmi.edu

L. Atanelov (ed.), *Resident's Handbook of Medical Quality and Safety*, DOI 10.1007/978-3-319-24190-6_34

Installation of R

One word of advice in working with R is that it may not be intuitive, which includes the installing of the program. RStudio is freeware that would make programming easy. Download the base program from http://www.r-project.org/. This is a prerequisite for running RStudio, which can be downloaded from here: http://www.rstudio.com/products/RStudio/. From here, you can install the program using the computer's installer.

Load Data (e.g., from Excel Sheet, Text Document, etc.)

Reading an Excel File [1]

Reading and Excel file can be simple. The first step would to be to save your Excel file as a csv file. Then, use the read.csv function with the filename in quotations, as below. Each cell inside such data file is separated by a special character, which usually is a comma. The first row of the data file should contain the column names instead of the actual data. Here is a sample of the expected format:

```
Col1,Col2,Col3
100,a1,b1
200,a2,b2
300,a3,b3
>mydata=read.csv("mydata.csv") #read csv file
>mydata
 Col1 Col2 Col3
   1 100  a1  b1
   2 200  a2  b2
   3 300  a3  b3
```

Note that we can also create a text file of a table and separate it by commas. After we copy and paste the data above in a file named "mydata.csv" with a text editor, we can read the data with the function read.csv.

R Interface/Console

Open up the RStudio program. You will find that there is a command prompt. Commands that are typed into the command prompt are called expressions. The interpreter will read the expression and return an output or an error. Examples of expressions and commands that you can place into the command prompt and the consequent results are:

```
>1+1
[1]2
>2*3
[1]6
```

The [1] *means that the returned value is interpreted as a vector and that there the first index of the first item is 1. There are many objects within R and can be defined by assigning objects and defining them as vectors, data frames, lists,* etc.

a <-as.data.frame([1:10], defines the numbers 1:10 and makes a data frame and calls it "a." Other useful operators include the "$" sign which allows you to extract elements of a data set. For example, in the example above for "mydata," entering mydata$Col1 will give you all the values of just Col1. The tilde operator "~" is used to separate parts of a model formula and is useful for statistics as will be demonstrated in multiple examples later in this chapter. Another really useful tool is the "for" loop. We will provide a brief example here, as for loops may be useful in going through individual elements of a data frame, performing an operator on it, and printing a value. Let us say we have a list of values, 1–5, called "c." If we wanted to find the square of each loop through c, the for() loop *will loop through 1–5 and take the square. Here is an example of that loop:*

```
> c <-(1:5)
> for(i in 1:(length(c))){
+ print(i^2)}
[1] 1
[1] 4
[1] 9
[1] 16
[1] 25
```

After the "for" and in between the parentheses is the formula that tells the for() loop what data to loop through. After the brackets, you can give the instructions as to what you would like the for() loop to do. Also note the difference between the above and the example presented below:

```
> c <-(2:5)
> for (i in c){
+ print(i^2)}
[1] 4
[1] 9
[1] 16
[1] 25
```

Finally, throughout this chapter and in R, having a "#" sign can allow one to annotate lines of code without having that annotation influence the code at all.

Analyzing Data Through R

Continuous Data (e.g., Grouped Data, e.g., Age of Group 1 versus Group 2)

Comparing continuous data involves the comparison of two groups that can take any value along a range. For example, age within a group, heights in a group of human beings, and chemical concentrations. These are usually measured. Discrete or non-continuous data is usually counted, like the number of people in a class or study.

Analysis of Continuous Data: Power Analysis

When designing an experiment, it's often helpful to know how much data you need to get a statistically significant sample (or the maximum significance of results that can be calculated from a given amount of data). These two questions can be easily answered in R with the power t test command. Let's assume that you have 120 patients in a study where you want to find a significant difference in the means of 60 patients randomized to a test vs. *60 patients to placebo. Let's also assume that the power of the test is 0.95, and the standard deviation of the population is 11.2:*

```
> power.t.test(power=0.95, sig.level=.05, sd=11.2, n=60)
   Two-sample t test power calculation
           n = 60
       delta = 7.432047
          sd = 11.2
   sig.level = 0.05
       power = 0.95
 alternative = two.sided
NOTE: n is number in *each* group
```

This states that the difference in means between the two groups would need to be at least 7.43 (delta) to be significant.

Descriptive Stats/Visualization

R provides a wide range of functions for obtaining summary statistics. The following functions and packages are extremely useful for obtaining a look at means, medians, standard deviations, etc. *For example, say you want to look at a set of numbers and wanted to quickly see what numbers lie in various quartiles. Let's take the numbers 1–25 as an easy example:*

```
> a <-c(1:25)
> a
 [1] 1 2 3 4 5 6 7 8 9 10 11 12 13 14 15 16 17 18 19 20
21 22 23 24 25
> summary(a)
```

```
   Min. 1st Qu.  Median    Mean 3rd Qu.    Max.
      1       7      13      13      19      25
```

This shows the minimum, first quartile, median, mean, third quartile, and maximum values for the data set.

Alternatively, one can use the Hmisc package after downloading it:

```
>library(Hmisc)
> describe(a)
a
      n missing unique    Mean    .05    .10    .25    .50    .75
.90    .95
     25       0     25      13    2.2    3.4    7.0   13.0   19.0   22.6
23.8
lowest :  1  2  3  4  5, highest: 21 22 23 24 25
```

Or the pastecs package:

```
>library(pastecs)
> stat.desc(mydata)
```

which gives min max, range, sum, median, mean, SE.mean, CI.mean, var, std.dev, coef.var [2].

Comparison of Two Groups: T tests

The student's t test can be easily manipulated like the above to obtain any of the parameters: n, delta, sig.level, or power. *You would have to provide at least four of the parameters. When wanting to calculate a p value to evaluate whether or not the mean of the experimental data is close to what the experimenter expected (null hypothesis), one can use the following* [3]:

```
t.test(x, y = NULL,
       alternative = c("two.sided", "less", "greater"),
       mu = 0, paired = FALSE, var.equal = FALSE,
       conf.level = 0.95, ...)
## S3 method for class 'formula'
t.test(formula, data, subset, na.action, ...)
```

For our example of numbers 1–25 above, if we wanted to calculate the p value of the t test, comparing that mean with another sample (mu, of 10):

```
t.test(a, mu=10)
   One Sample t-test
data:  a
t = 2.0381, df = 24, p-value = 0.05271
alternative hypothesis: true mean is not equal to 10
95 percent confidence interval:
 9.962024 16.037976
sample estimates:
mean of x
     13
```

This states that the differences in mean is not significant, as the p value is greater than 0.05.

Nonparametrics

In statistics, there are other tests that can analyze whether or not two data sets are statistically identical, based on the format of the data. Some tests that people most use for non-normally distributed data are the Mann–Whitney U test, the Wilcoxon Rank Sum Test, and the Kruskal–Wallis test. These tests with some examples are included below:

```
# independent 2-group Mann-Whitney U Test
wilcox.test(y~A)
```

where y is numeric and A is a binary factor. The "~" is separating the two parts of the formula, as it will for other formulas and examples below.

The mtcars data that is included with R offers a nice data set to be able to play with and demonstrate these tests. Once you have downloaded RStudio, view the data set:

>View(mtcars) #this should bring up a viewable form of the data set.

(See Table 1)

```
> wilcox.test(mpg ~ am, data=mtcars)
Wilcoxon rank sum test with continuity correction
data:  mpg by am
W = 42, p-value = 0.001871
alternative hypothesis: true location shift is not equal to 0
```

TABLE 1 Table of the "mtcars" dataset

	row.names	mpg	cyl	disp	hp	drat	wt	qsec	vs	am	gear	carb
1	Mazda RX4	21.0	6	160.0	110	3.90	2.620	16.46	0	1	4	4
2	Mazda RX4 Wag	21.0	6	160.0	110	3.90	2.875	17.02	0	1	4	4
3	Datsun 710	22.8	4	108.0	93	3.85	2.320	18.61	1	1	4	1
4	Hornet 4 Drive	21.4	6	258.0	110	3.08	3.215	19.44	1	0	3	1
5	Hornet Sportabout	18.7	8	360.0	175	3.15	3.440	17.02	0	0	3	2
6	Valiant	18.1	6	225.0	105	2.76	3.460	20.22	1	0	3	1
7	Duster 360	14.3	8	360.0	245	3.21	3.570	15.84	0	0	3	4
8	Merc 240D	24.4	4	146.7	62	3.69	3.190	20.00	1	0	4	2
9	Merc 230	22.8	4	140.8	95	3.92	3.150	22.90	1	0	4	2
10	Merc 280	19.2	6	167.6	123	3.92	3.440	18.30	1	0	4	4
11	Merc 280C	17.8	6	167.6	123	3.92	3.440	18.90	1	0	4	4
12	Merc 450SE	16.4	8	275.8	180	3.07	4.070	17.40	0	0	3	3

13	Merc 450SL	17.3	8	275.8	180	3.07	3.730	17.60	0	0	3	3
14	Merc 450SLC	15.2	8	275.8	180	3.07	3.780	18.00	0	0	3	3
15	Cadillac Fleetwood	10.4	8	472.0	205	2.93	5.250	17.98	0	0	3	4
16	Lincoln Continental	10.4	8	460.0	215	3.00	5.424	17.82	0	0	3	4
17	Chrysler Imperial	14.7	8	440.0	230	3.23	5.345	17.42	0	0	3	4
18	Fiat 128	32.4	4	78.7	66	4.08	2.200	19.47	1	1	4	1
19	Honda Civic	30.4	4	75.7	52	4.93	1.615	18.52	1	1	4	2
20	Toyota Corolla	33.9	4	71.1	65	4.22	1.835	19.90	1	1	4	1
21	Toyota Corona	21.5	4	120.1	97	3.70	2.465	20.01	1	0	3	1
22	Dodge Challenger	15.5	8	318.0	150	2.76	3.520	16.87	0	0	3	2

(continued)

Table 1 (continued)

	row.names	mpg	cyl	disp	hp	drat	wt	qsec	vs	am	gear	carb
23	AMC Javelin	15.2	8	304.0	150	3.15	3.435	17.30	0	0	3	2
24	Camaro Z28	13.3	8	350.0	245	3.73	3.840	15.41	0	0	3	4
25	Pontiac Firebird	19.2	8	400.0	175	3.08	3.845	17.05	0	0	3	2
26	Fiat X1-9	27.3	4	79.0	66	4.08	1.935	18.90	1	1	4	1
27	Porsche 914-2	26.0	4	120.3	91	4.43	2.140	16.70	0	1	5	2
28	Lotus Europa	30.4	4	95.1	113	3.77	1.513	16.90	1	1	5	2
29	Ford Pantera L	15.8	8	351.0	264	4.22	3.170	14.50	0	1	5	4
30	Ferrari Dino	19.7	6	145.0	175	3.62	2.770	15.50	0	1	5	6
31	Maserati Bora	15.0	8	301.0	335	3.54	3.570	14.60	0	1	5	8
32	Volvo 142E	21.4	4	121.0	109	4.11	2.780	18.60	1	1	4	2

The mpg column gives the miles per gallon while the am column denotes the transmission (automatic=0, manual=1). To decide whether or not these two populations are statistically identical, one can use the Mann–Whitney U Test, where A is a binary factor

```
Warning message:
In wilcox.test.default(x = c(21.4, 18.7, 18.1, 14.3, 24.4, 22.8, :
  cannot compute exact p-value with ties
```

In this example, there is a difference between the two data sets, as denoted by the low p value:

```
# independent 2-group Mann-Whitney U Test
wilcox.test(y,x) # where y and x are numeric
wilcox.test(y,x, correct=FALSE)
> wilcox.test(c(1:5),c(6:10), correct=FALSE)
    Wilcoxon rank sum test
data:  c(1:5) and c(6:10)
W = 0, p-value = 0.007937
alternative hypothesis: true location shift is not equal to 0
```

The p value is less than 0.05, which means we can safely say that the two groups are statistically different.

A similar test can be done on the mtcars data set as well for analyzing data that are identical. To determine whether or not the mpg and the hp (horsepower) data are identical, one can use the following:

```
# dependent 2-group Wilcoxon Signed Rank Test
wilcox.test(y1,y2,paired=TRUE) # where y1 and y2 are numeric
wilcox.test(mtcars$mpg, mtcars$hp, paired=TRUE)
    Wilcoxon signed rank test with continuity correction
data:  mtcars$mpg and mtcars$hp
V = 0, p-value = 8.338e-07
alternative hypothesis: true location shift is not equal to 0
Warning message:
In wilcox.test.default(mtcars$mpg, mtcars$hp, paired = TRUE) :
  cannot compute exact p-value with ties
```

The Kruskal–Wallis Test is a test to evaluate whether or not two or more samples come from the same distribution. This is very useful for samples that may be of different length and when comparing more than two groups. Let us look at the air quality data set provided by R. If one wanted to see if Ozone and Month come from the same distribution, one can run the following code:

```
# Kruskal Wallis Test One Way Anova by Ranks
kruskal.test(y~A) # where y1 is numeric and A is a factor
> head(airquality)
  Ozone Solar.R Wind Temp Month Day
1    41     190  7.4   67     5   1
2    36     118  8.0   72     5   2
3    12     149 12.6   74     5   3
4    18     313 11.5   62     5   4
5    NA      NA 14.3   56     5   5
6    28      NA 14.9   66     5   6
>kruskal.test(Ozone ~ Month,data=airquality)
      Kruskal-Wallis rank sum test
data: Ozone by Month
Kruskal-Wallis chi-squared=29.267,df=4,p-value=6.901e-06
#Our p-value denotes that these do not come from the same distribution.
```

Several Groups: ANOVA and ANCOVA

One-way analysis of variance:

Using the InsectSprays data frame included in R, one can run a one way ANOVA by the following. ANOVA is a method to compare means across two or more groups. Below is an example of discrete data, but the same analysis can be performed for non-discrete or continuous data as well. If one wanted to compare the one-way analysis of variance for count and spray, one can run the following code:

```
> head(InsectSprays) #to view part of the dataframe
  count spray
1    10     A
2     7     A
3    20     A
4    14     A
5    14     A
6    12     A
> aov(count~spray, data=InsectSprays) ->aov
> summary(aov)
```

```
          Df Sum Sq Mean Sq F value Pr(>F)
spray      5   2669   533.8    34.7 <2e-16 ***
Residuals 66   1015    15.4
---
Signif. codes:  0 '***' 0.001 '**' 0.01 '*' 0.05 '.' 0.1 ' ' 1
```

where the p value is Pr(>F), and the F value tells us how far away we are from the hypothesis that:"we cannot distinguish between error and treatment (treatment is irrelevant)" [3,4]. *A big F implies that treatment does not matter. The p value is low in this case, indicating that the means are statistically different.*

ANCOVA

ANOVA, the analysis of variance, is a way to test the equality of the means of different groups. There are instances when there will be certain factors that will confound the relationships between sets of data. The regression of ANOVA can be extrapolated to include other variables that may influence a certain outcome. These are known as covariates, and determining whether or not a covariate has a significant effect on an outcome is known as ANCOVA or analysis of covariance. ANCOVA can be a complicated topic, and for further information and detail on running ANCOVA, the reader is directed to an excellent book on this complicated topic, Discovering Statistics Using R by Andy Field et al.

As a brief example, let us consider a simple example of low, medium, and high levels of Drug X that enhances mental functioning and test scores. There are a myriad of covariates that could potentially affect test scores, including intelligence, hours of sleep, previous experience in a subject, etc. *Let us choose IQ as a covariate based on the following data:*

```
dose <-c(rep(1,5), rep(3,9), rep(4,12), rep(2, 4))
grade <-c(rep(1, 10), rep(2,10), rep(3,10))
intelligence <-c(100, 101, 100, 101, 102, 103, 101, 104, 105,
100, 120, 121, 120, 121, 125, 122, 125, 120, 120, 125, 140, 141,
140, 141, 145, 150, 140, 140, 142, 141)
experiment <-data.frame(dose, grade, intelligence)
```

See Table 2.

TABLE 2 Table of Drug X, Grade, and Intelligence

	Dose	Grade	Intelligence
1	1	1	100
2	1	1	101
3	1	1	100
4	1	1	101
5	1	1	102
6	3	1	103
7	3	1	101
8	3	1	104
9	3	1	105
10	3	1	100
11	3	2	120
12	3	2	121
13	3	2	120
14	3	2	121
15	4	2	125
16	4	2	122
17	4	2	125
18	4	2	120
19	4	2	120
20	4	2	125
21	4	3	140
22	4	3	141
23	4	3	140
24	4	3	141
25	4	3	145

(continued)

Table 2 (continued)

	Dose	Grade	Intelligence
26	4	3	150
27	2	3	140
28	2	3	140
29	2	3	142
30	2	3	141

Let us try to determine if intelligence is a covariate that significantly influences test scores. One would first test the interaction of dose on grade, intelligence on grade, and whether or not there is an interaction between dose and intelligence:

```
>mod1<-aov(grade~dose*intelligence,data=experiment)
> summary(mod1)
                  Df Sum Sq Mean Sq  F value   Pr(>F)
dose               1  4.015   4.015  300.233 8.43e-16 ***
intelligence       1 15.622  15.622 1168.184  < 2e-16 ***
dose:intelligence  1  0.016   0.016    1.188    0.286
Residuals         26  0.348   0.013
---
Signif. codes:  0 '***' 0.001 '**' 0.01 '*' 0.05 '.' 0.1 ' ' 1
```

This shows a significant interaction between effect of dose and intelligence but no interaction together (dose: intelligence). Furthermore, a quicker model would be to test for differences in slope. Differences in slope in ANCOVA denote different effects on the dependent variable and are suggestive of the presence of an interacting covariate:

```
mod2 <-aov(grade~dose+intelligence, data=experiment)
> summary(mod2)
             Df Sum Sq Mean Sq F value   Pr(>F)
dose          1  4.015   4.015   298.2 4.07e-16 ***
intelligence  1 15.622  15.622  1160.1  < 2e-16 ***
Residuals    27  0.364   0.013
---
Signif. codes:  0 '***' 0.001 '**' 0.01 '*' 0.05 '.' 0.1 ' ' 1
```

Now check to see if removing the interaction affects the fit of the model:

```
> anova(mod1,mod2)
Analysis of Variance Table
Model 1: grade ~ dose * intelligence
Model 2: grade ~ dose + intelligence
  Res.Df     RSS Df Sum of Sq      F Pr(>F)
1     26 0.34769
2     27 0.36357 -1 -0.015885 1.1879 0.2858
```

This shows that the interaction (intelligence and dose) does not significantly affect the fit of the model, given the high p value [5,6].

Correlations

Sometimes the question is whether or not two continuous variables are correlated. Such questions can involve issues like "is there a correlation between increase in exercise in 6th graders and test scores?" When we increase a variable, how much does the other variable increase and by how much (nutshell)? The cor() function is a powerful tool in R to be able to calculate this. Let us look at an example from the mtcars data set to see if there is a correlation between mpg for cars and their weight based on the Pearson calculation:

```
cor(mtcars$mpg, mtcars$wt, method="pearson")
[1] -0.8676594
```

Note that one can also calculate a Spearman and Kendall R value by setting a method equal to "spearman" or "kendall," respectively. To determine if this correlation is significant, use cor.test:

```
cor.test(mtcars$mpg, mtcars$wt, method="pearson")
   Pearson's product-moment correlation
data:  mtcars$mpg and mtcars$wt
t = -9.559, df = 30, p-value = 1.294e-10
alternative hypothesis: true correlation is not equal to 0
```

```
95 percent confidence interval:
 -0.9338264 -0.7440872
sample estimates:
       cor
-0.8676594
```

It appears that the correlation of miles per gallon and their weight has a significant correlation with an R of –0.868.

Regressions

Let's take the above example and perform a regression. What is the regression between the weight of cars and their miles per gallon?

```
> reg = lm(mtcars$wt~mtcars$mpg)
> reg
Call:
lm(formula = mtcars$wt ~ mtcars$mpg)
Coefficients:
(Intercept)  mtcars$mpg
    6.0473      -0.1409
```

Here, the y-intercept of the linear regression is 6.0473 and the slope is –0.1409. Note that regression could also be run on different variables to see how several independent variables together impact the dependent variable, e.g., *how altitude and percentage humidity affect the weight of coffee beans produced. See implementation of a different example using Poisson model below. Adding extra independent variables is done by the "+" sign.*

Non-continuous Data

There are different tests for calculating statistical significance for discrete data (e.g., color of tea, green vs. black; sex, male or female; car model, Toyota, Nissan, Ford, etc.).

Power Analysis

When it comes to determining the relationship between two variables, one has a myriad of options. Two popular and useful tests are the Fisher exact test (most used for two-by-two contingency tables) and chi-square test (for larger sets of data). In these cases, a high p value implies that the groups are independent of each other while a low p value implies that the groups being compared are not independent. Let us take an example of the original Fisher exact test. Dr. Fisher (from the Fisher exact test) had an acquaintance, Dr. Muriel Bristo, who claimed to be able to detect whether tea or milk was added first to her cup of tea. Was the tea put in first or the milk? One can generate this scenario by the following code from stat.ethz.ch.

Fisher Exact Test:

```
> TeaTasting <-
+   matrix(c(3, 1, 1, 3),
+        nrow = 2,
+        dimnames = list(Guess = c("Milk", "Tea"),
+                        Truth = c("Milk", "Tea")))
> fisher.test(TeaTasting, alternative = "greater")
   Fisher's Exact Test for Count Data
data:  TeaTasting
p-value = 0.2429
alternative hypothesis: true odds ratio is greater than 1
95 percent confidence interval:
 0.3135693       Inf
sample estimates:
odds ratio
  6.408309
```

An association could not be established. Here is the complete code with all options:

```
fisher.test(x, y = NULL, workspace = 200000, hybrid = FALSE,
            control = list(), or = 1, alternative = "two.sided",
            conf.int = TRUE, conf.level = 0.95,
            simulate.p.value = FALSE, B = 2000)
```

The "alternative" argument must be one of "two-sided," "greater," or "less" for Fisher exact test, as in "the alternative hypothesis is 'greater' or 'less'" [7].

Chi-Square Test:

The chi-square test is usually used to evaluate if the frequency in a population is different than the expected frequency. Take this example in a hypothetical class of people enrolled in an English class; their attractiveness and scores at the end of the class were tabulated:

```
> ClassGrades <-matrix(c(1:15), nrow = 3, dimnames = list(Appearance = c("ugly", "normal", "attractive"), Grade = c("A", "B", "C", "D", "F")))
>View(ClassGrades)
```

See Table 3.

```
> chisq.test(ClassGrades)
   Pearson's Chi-squared test
data:  ClassGrades
X-squared = 0.7362, df = 8, p-value = 0.9994
```

It is likely that the two variables are independent given the high p value.

Descriptive Stats/Visualization

Much of the functions above like summary() and describe() will work for discrete data as well:

```
summary(ClassGrades)
      A          B          C          D           F
 Min.  :1.0  Min.  :4.0  Min.  :7.0  Min.  :10.0  Min.  :13.0
```

TABLE 3 Table of grade by attractiveness of the student

	row.names	A	B	C	D	E
1	Ugly	1	4	7	10	13
2	Normal	2	5	8	11	14
3	Attractive	3	6	9	12	15

```
1st Qu.:1.5   1st Qu.:4.5   1st Qu.:7.5   1st Qu.:10.5   1st Qu.:13.5
Median :2.0   Median :5.0   Median :8.0   Median :11.0   Median :14.0
Mean   :2.0   Mean   :5.0   Mean   :8.0   Mean   :11.0   Mean   :14.0
3rd Qu.:2.5   3rd Qu.:5.5   3rd Qu.:8.5   3rd Qu.:11.5   3rd Qu.:14.5
Max.   :3.0   Max.   :6.0   Max.   :9.0   Max.   :12.0   Max.   :15.0
```

Frequencies and Cross Tables

The table function in R provides a great tool for evaluating the frequencies that a specific number shows up in a list. This is useful when looking at how much times a given count shows up:

```
> a <- rep(c(NA, 1/0:3), 10)
> table(a)
a
0.333333333333333              0.5                1              Inf
               10               10               10               10
```

One can also perform a two-way cross tabulation through the CrossTable() function in R to generate a table of chi-square and Fisher tests, Pearson correlation, etc.

Correlations

For discrete data, it is appropriate to use the Spearman correlation coefficient to calculate correlations between sets of data. The cloth data set will be used in this case and also comes as part of R. In the R data frame, x is the length of a roll of cloth and y is the number of flaws found in the roll:

```
> head(cloth)
     x y
1 1.22 1
2 1.70 4
```

```
3 2.71  5
4 3.71 14
5 3.72  7
6 3.75  9
> cor.test(cloth$x,cloth$y, method="spearman")
   Spearman's rank correlation rho
data:  cloth$x and cloth$y
S = 2323.999, p-value = 0.0005918
alternative hypothesis: true rho is not equal to 0
sample estimates:
     rho
0.5740471
Warning message:
In cor.test.default(cloth$x, cloth$y, method = "spearman"):
  Cannot compute exact p-value with ties
```

The Spearman's rank correlation rho is 0.57401 with a significant p value.

Regressions: Poisson Regression

The Institute for Digital Research and Education at UCLA has a great tutorial on using the Poisson distribution to perform a regression on data [9]. To generate a Poisson regression examining the number of awards vs. "program" or "math," one can use the generalized linear model function (glm) and specifying "poisson" as the "family" [9]. The main question being answered below is: "*how is program or math (here also known as predictor variables) influencing number of awards (the outcome variable)?*" *We are also assuming here that the data below follows a Poisson distribution:*

View(head(p, 30)) #this gives the first 30 rows of the p data set

See Table 4.

> summary(m1 <- glm(num_awards ~ prog + math, family = "poisson", data = p))

Call:

TABLE 4 Table of the first 30 rows of the "p" dataset

	id	num_awards	prog	math
1	45	0	Vocational	41
2	108	0	General	41
3	15	0	Vocational	44
4	67	0	Vocational	42
5	153	0	Vocational	40
6	51	0	General	42
7	164	0	Vocational	46
8	133	0	Vocational	40
9	2	0	Vocational	33
10	53	0	Vocational	46
11	1	0	Vocational	40
12	128	0	Academic	38
13	16	0	Vocational	44
14	106	0	Vocational	37
15	89	0	Vocational	40
16	134	0	General	39
17	19	0	General	43
18	145	0	Vocational	38
19	11	0	Academic	45
20	117	0	Vocational	39
21	109	0	General	42
22	12	0	Vocational	45
23	37	0	Vocational	40
24	69	0	Vocational	40
25	43	0	Academic	43

(continued)

Table 4 (continued)

	id	num_awards	prog	math
26	196	0	Academic	49
27	36	1	General	44
28	155	1	General	46
29	6	0	Academic	46
30	4	1	Academic	41

```
glm(formula = num_awards ~ prog + math, family = "poisson", data = p)
Deviancc Residuals:
    Min       1Q   Median       3Q      Max
-2.1840  -0.9003  -0.5891   0.3948   2.9539
Coefficients:
             Estimate Std. Error z value Pr(>|z|)
(Intercept) -5.578057   0.676823  -8.242   <2e-16 ***
prog         0.123273   0.163261   0.755     0.45
math         0.086121   0.009586   8.984   <2e-16 ***
---
Signif. codes:  0 '***' 0.001 '**' 0.01 '*' 0.05 '.' 0.1 ' ' 1
(Dispersion parameter for poisson family taken to be 1)
    Null deviance: 287.67  on 199  degrees of freedom
Residual deviance: 203.45  on 197  degrees of freedom
AIC: 385.51
Number of Fisher Scoring iterations: 6
```

Above we are provided with an estimate of the response variable (number of awards) for each predictor variable (program or math). The glm() function returns the estimate of the intercept, standard error, z value, and Pr value of the regression. We see that there is a significant effect of math. You may be wondering why we used lm and glm for regressions, and the above example is a perfect reason why. The math behind lm() vs. glm() is somewhat complicated, but for our purposes, glm, the generalized linear model, allows us to fit other distributions to allow for a prediction. As above, we used a Poisson distribution, but one can use gamma, inverse Gaussian, or quasi distributions. Fitting an ordinary linear regression with both lm() and glm() should give the same results.

How To Write a File

When writing a file, one can use the "write.table" function. One has to be sure that the data is already in a data frame or matrix:

```
write.table(x, file = "", append = FALSE, quote = TRUE,
sep = " ",
        eol = "\n", na = "NA", dec = ".", row.names = TRUE,
                col.names = TRUE, qmethod = c("escape",
"double"),
          fileEncoding = "")
```

or

```
write.csv(...)
write.csv2(...)
```

for csv files.

For example, a good exercise is to try to write the mtcars data frame into an Excel file for viewing and manipulation:

```
write.table(mtcars, file="mtcars.xls", sep=",")
```

Then try to open the file in Excel. Excel will ask you what the delimiter is and you can specify "comma." The data should open in Excel.

Six Sigma Functions

Six Sigma is the use of statistical software to improve processes within companies and institutions. Six sigma requires the use of statistical software which R provides. Many books have been written on the subject. The basic design of the Six Sigma philosophy is Design, Measure, Analyze, Improve, and Control. After downloading the Six Sigma package in R, there are tons of possibilities and formulas to use to answer questions about streamlining processes. For instance, there is a loss of function analysis within the Six Sigma package. The reader is directed to the table below of functions, taken from Six Sigma with R, Statistical Engineering for Process Improvement by Cano et al. [8]

Argument	**Description**
lfa.data	Data frame with data sample
lfa.ctq	Name of field in data frame containing data
lfa.Delta	Process tolerance
lfa.Y0	Process target
lfa.L0	Cost of poor quality at tolerance limit
lfa.size	Number of items to calculate total loss in a group
lfa.output	String with type of output: "text," "plot," "both"
lfa.sub	Subtitle of graphic output

The ss.rr function in the Six Sigma package is also a very convenient tool to be able to get quick plots and an ANOVA of your data. After running it you get an output of the ANOVA table, variance details, and bar charts [8].

> ss.rr(var, part, appr, data, main, sub)

In terms of the "analyze" part of the Six Sigma paradigm, many of the functions are already included with the base package of R, including boxplot(). One can even calculate binominal distributions for given parameters. For instance, if one wanted to calculate the probability of obtaining five or fewer defects with an n of 120 and a rate of 2% defects:

>pbinom(5, 120, 0.02)

Much of the statistical analyses and functions are again part of the base package of R. However, there are Six Sigma functions that are part of the package and are useful for higher-level analyses. They are included for completeness below [8].

Function	**Task**
ss.ceDiag	Cause-and-effect diagram
ss.pMap	Process map
ss.lfa	Loss function analysis

Function	Task
ss.lfa	Computes loss function value
ss.rr	Gage R and R study
ss.study.ca	Capability analysis study
ss.ca.cp	Capability index
ss.ca.cpk	Corrected capability index
ss.ca.yield	Computes yield of a process
ss.ci	Confidence interval for mean and normality test

Online References for R

http://www.ats.ucla.edu/stat/r/seminars/intro.R
http://www.statmethods.net/stATS/index.html
http://www.r-tutor.com/
http://cran.us.r-project.org/
http://stackoverflow.com/

If you have any questions about the information covered in this chapter or other medical safety and quality improvement-related topics, please contact us at http://www.medicalqualityandsafetyforum.com. The website will also provide a forum where you can ask specific questions about your safety and medical quality improvement projects or mentor upcoming medical quality leaders.

Additional Resources

1. Yau, Chi. "Data Import." *R Tutorial: An R Introduction to Statistics*. N.p., n.d. Web. 21 Aug. 2014
2. Adler, Joseph. *R in a Nutshell.* Sebastopol: O'Reilly Media, Inc. 2010. Book

3. Grosjean, Philippe, and Frederic Ibanez. "Package 'pastecs'." (n.d.): n. pag. 3 Feb. 2014. Web. 8 Aug. 2014. http://cran.r-project.org/web/packages/pastecs/pastecs.pdf
4. http://stat.ethz.ch/education/semesters/as2013/anova/ANOVA_how_to_do.pdf
5. http://stat.ethz.ch/R-manual/R-patched/library/stats/html/fisher.test.html
6. http://www.ats.ucla.edu/stat/r/dae/poissonreg.htm
7. R in Ecology and Evolution: Comparing two regression slopes by means of an ANCOVA. (n.d.). Retrieved September 9, 2014
8. Field, A., & Miles, J. (2012). *Discovering statistics using R*. London: Sage. R documentation: http://www.r-project.org/

References

1. Yau C. "Data import." R tutorial an R introduction to statistics. N.p., n.d. Web. 21 Aug 2014.
2. Grossjean P, Ibanez F. Package 'pastecs'. (n.d.): n. pag. 3 Feb 2014. Web. 8 Aug 2014. http://cran.r-project.org/web/packages/pastecs/pastecs.pdf
3. Adler J. R in a nutshell. Sebastopol: O'Reilly Media; 2010. Book.
4. http://stat.ethz.ch/education/semesters/as2013/anova/ANOVA_how_to_do.pdf
5. R in ecology and evolution: comparing two regression slopes by means of an ANCOVA. (n.d.). Retrieved September 9, 2014.
6. Field A, Miles J. Discovering statistics using R. London: Sage; 2012.
7. Martin M. http://stat.ethz.ch/R-manual/R-patched/library/stats/html/fisher.test.html
8. Cano E, Moguerza J, Redchuk A. Six sigma with R: statistical engineering for process improvement. New York: Springer Science and Business Media; 2012. Print.
9. http://www.ats.ucla.edu/stat/r/dae/poissonreg.htm

ERRATUM TO

Implementing Early Rehabilitation in the ICU to Improve Patient Outcomes

DMAIC Phase: *Control*

Ibtehal Kimawi and Dale M. Needham

L. Atanelov (ed.), Resident's Handbook of Medical Quality and Safety, DOI 10.1007/978-3-319-24190-6_14

DOI 10.1007/978-3-319-24190-6_35

The print and online versions of the book contain an error in a contributor's name. The corrections to this name are given as "Dale M. Needham" on the following pages:

1. On page xii in the table of contents
2. On page xvi in the contributor's list
3. On page 109 in Chapter 14 titled "Implementing Early Rehabilitation in the ICU to Improve Patient Outcomes"

The updated online version of the original chapter can be found under http://dx.doi.org/10.1007/978-3-319-24190-6_14

L. Atanelov (ed.), Resident's Handbook of Medical Quality and Safety, DOI 10.1007/978-3-319-24190-6_35

Index

A

Absolute risk reduction (ARR), 335
Academic medical center's quality improvement programs, 37–39
Accountability, 4, 5
Accountable care organization, 6
Accreditation Association for Ambulatory Healthcare (AAAHC), 12
Accreditation Council for Graduate Medical Education (ACGME) program, 38, 52
Active listening, 223, 226–228
Activity network diagram, 249–250
Acute care therapy, 118–127
ADC. *See* Automated dispensing cabinets (ADC)
Adverse event reports, 45
Affinity diagram, 236–237
Agency of Healthcare Reform and Quality (AHRQ), 262–263
AIPSQ. *See* Armstrong Institute for Patient Safety and Quality (AIPSQ)
American Academy of Physical Medicine and Rehabilitation, 113
American Thoracic Society, 113
Analysis of covariance (ANCOVA), 348, 375–378
Analysis of variance (ANOVA) test, 137, 321, 324, 325, 374–375
A3 problem-solving tool, 290, 291, 302–308
Armstrong Institute for Patient Safety and Quality (AIPSQ), 52
ARR. *See* Absolute risk reduction (ARR)
Ask Me 3 Program, 227–228
Assist residency training programs, 52
Attributable risk, 335
Automated dispensing cabinets (ADC), 138–142

B

Baclofen pump therapy, 158–160
Balance arrow, 311–312
Barriers scale, 62
Belbin's team roles, 259

L. Atanelov (ed.), *Resident's Handbook of Medical Quality and Safety*, DOI 10.1007/978-3-319-24190-6

Benefit effort matrix tool, 315–317
Bias, 175, 179, 336
Bibliographic citation managers, 162–163
Bonnie's approach, 322–323
Boolean operators, 153–154
Bowtie model, 17
Brainstorming, 235
Brainwriting techniques, 235–236
Briefings, 223

C
Callout, 222
Case–control study, 333
Catheter Associated Urinary Tract Infection (CAUTI) project, 129–132
Cause-and-effect diagram. *See* Fishbone diagram
CBA. *See* Cost-benefit analysis (CBA)
Centers for Medicare and Medicaid Services (CMS), 14
Certified practitioners, 271
CFA. *See* Confirmatory factor analysis (CFA)
Checkback, 222
Check sheets, 239–240
Chi-square test, 380, 381
Clinical Learning Environment Review (CLER) program, 38, 43–44
Clinical outcomes, 4–5, 353–354
Clinical studies, 172–176, 179
Closed populations, 334
CMS. *See* Centers for Medicare and Medicaid Services (CMS)
Cognitive ergonomics, 22
Cognitive walk-through, 24
Cohort study, 333
Communication healthcare tools, 220–231
Confirmatory factor analysis (CFA), 360
Conflict management, 229–230
Contextual inquiry, 24
Continuous quality improvement, 4
Cost-benefit analysis (CBA), 247
Cost-benefit matrix, 288–289, 296
Crew resource management (CRM), 226
Critical appraisal, 166
Critical to quality (CTQ), 286
Culture of safety, 44–45
Customer feedback, 285
CUS words, 230, 231

D
Data collection, 342–343
Data mining, 30–31
Defects per million opportunities (DPMO), 318, 319
Define, Measure, Analyze, Improve, and Control (DMAIC), 66
  acute care therapy services, 119–125
  A3 problem-solving tool, 290, 291, 302–308
  certified practitioners, 271
  early-in-day discharge, 94–98
  global immunization core measure, 105–107
  idea generation process, 189–192
  idea selection process, 189–192
  patient discharge communication, 71–79
  patients mobility, 59–64
  post-hospital syndrome, 271–275

quality improvement, 189–192, 268–271
Six Sigma methodology, 268–271, 323–324, 326–327
smoking cessation in pregnancy, 83–85
stat medication process, 137–142
Delphi technique, 246–247
Deming cycle/wheel. *See* Plan, Do, Check, Act (PDCA) cycle
Descriptive statistics, 344, 345
DESC script, 231
DIAAT, 19–20
Didactic education, 46–47
Discharge Knowledge Assessment scores, 79
DMAIC. *See* Define, Measure, Analyze, Improve, and Control (DMAIC)
DPMO. *See* Defects per million opportunities (DPMO)

E

Early-in-day discharge, 92–99
EFA. *See* Exploratory factor analysis (EFA)
Eight Disciplines Problem Solving, 234–235
Electronic health records (EHR), 29–31
Electronic medical record (EMR), 5, 60, 173, 200
Embase, 153, 156, 157, 160
Empathy, 3
EndNote, 162
Epic MyChart (EMR), 79
EPIC systems, 31
Epidemiological risk factor model, 337
Epidemiological studies, 332–333
Evidence based medicine, 165–167
Exploratory factor analysis (EFA), 359–360

F

FA. *See* Functional analysis (FA)
Fall prevention, 341–349, 351
Federal Aviation Administration (FAA), 17–18
Field tags, 156–157
Filters, 161
Fishbone diagram, 77–78, 238–239, 280, 281, 317–318
Fisher's exact test, 137, 380
Flow chart, 244, 245
5 m model, 19
Foley placement, 130, 131
Force-field diagram/force-field analysis, 248
Functional analysis (FA), 17

G

Gantt chart, 250, 251
Global 8D, 234–235
Global immunization core measures 101–107

H

HAL. *See* Highest activity level (HAL)
Handoff, 222–223
Hawthorne effect, 79
HCAHPS scores, 70, 72
Health informatics, 30
Health Resources and Services Administration (HRSA), 13
Herzberg's motivation-hygiene theory, 259
Heuristic analysis, 24
HFE. *See* Human factors engineering (HFE)

Highest activity level (HAL), 272–275
High-reliability organization (HRO), 6–7, 226–227
Histogram, 241, 243
House Staff Patient Safety Quality Council (HPSQC), 38–39, 51–54, 102–108
HRO. *See* High-reliability organization (HRO)
HRSA. *See* Health Resources and Services Administration (HRSA)
Human factors engineering (HFE), 21–27
Hypothesis testing, 320, 344–347

I

ICU Recovery Network (IRN), 113
Idea generation process, 187–192
Idea selection process, 189–192
IHI. *See* Institute of Healthcare Improvement (IHI)
Improvement, 265–266
IMRAD format, 149
IMSAFE tool, 229
Incidence rate, 334
Information technology (IT), 53
In scope, 196–198
Institute of Healthcare Improvement (IHI), 12
Institute of Medicine (IOM), 12, 14
Institutional review board (IRB), 64, 112, 148
Intensive care unit (ICU), 111–113
Interrelationship diagram/relations diagram, 248–249
Interviews, 25
Intuitive systematic method, 179–183
IOM. *See* Institute of Medicine (IOM)
I PASS the BATON method, 223–225
IRB. *See* Institutional review board (IRB)
IRN. *See* ICU Recovery Network (IRN), 113
Ishikawa diagram. *See* Fishbone diagram

J

Johns Hopkins Highest Level of Mobility (JH-HLM) scale, 60
Johns Hopkins Hospital Medical Board, 51, 52
Joint Commission on Accreditation of Hospitals (JCAH), 11
Joint Commission on the Accreditation of Healthcare Organizations (JCAHO), 13

K

Kaizen rules, 296–298
Kanban, 317
Keywords *vs.* controlled vocabulary, 155–156
Kruskal–Wallis test, 369, 373–374

L

Leadership, 262
Lean six sigma, 301–327
Length of stay (LOS), 196
Linear regression, 348
LISREL, 360

Literature search, 153–163
Load data, 364–366

M
Macroergonomics, 22
Mann–Whitney U test, 369–373
Maslow hierarchy, 259–260
Measurement systems analysis (MSA), 305–306
Medical intensive care unit (MICU), 112
Medical quality, 5
Medical subject headings (MeSH), 155
MICU. *See* Medical intensive care unit (MICU)
Milgram experiment, 5–6
Minitab® box plot, 324, 326
Minitab® graph, 320, 322
Minitab® P-chart, 327
Morbidity and mortality (M&M) conference, 47–48
Motivation-hygiene theory, 259
MSA. *See* Measurement systems analysis (MSA)
Multidisciplinary rounds, 229
Multivariable regression, 61, 273

N
National Airspace System (NAS), 18
National Committee for Quality Assurance (NCQA), 14
National Patient Safety Foundation (NPSF), 12
National Practitioner Database (NPDB), 14
National Quality Forum (NQF), 14, 337
Necessary non-value added (NNVA) map, 310
Nominal group technique (NGT), 246
Non-value added (NVA) map, 309–310

O
Observational studies, 176–179
Occupational interests, 258
Occupational therapists (OT), 118
Odds ratio (OR), 335
Office of Human Right Protection (OHRP) guidance, 112
Open populations, 334
Out of scope, 196–198

P
Paper and pencil forms, 354
Pareto chart, 241–244
Patient discharge communication, 71–79
Patient safety, 10, 13, 42–44, 52, 65, 230, 336–338
Patients mobility, 57–68
PDCA cycle. *See* Plan, Do, Check, Act (PDCA) cycle
PHL. *See* Preliminary hazard list (PHL)
Physical ergonomics, 22
Physical therapists (PTs), 10, 118
Physician quality reporting system (PQRS), 3–4
PICO, 157–160
Plan, Do, Check, Act (PDCA) cycle, 61, 66–67, 129–132, 266–268, 273, 303–307, 309–314, 323–327
Plan-Do-Study-Act (PDSA) cycle, 267, 268
Poisson regression, 383–386
Post-hospital syndrome, 271–275
Power analysis, 367

PQRS. *See* Physician quality reporting system (PQRS)
Preliminary hazard list (PHL), 17
Prevalence, 87, 177, 182, 334
Preventative medicine, 6
Process capability, 318–320
Process flowchart, 278, 279
Project charter, 196, 205–208
Project management skills and visual tools, 234–252
Project scope, 198, 199, 212–217
Project scope creep, 196
Project Scope Guide, 196–198
Project selection, 203–205
Prototyping, 25
Publishing project, 147–151
PubMed, 58, 71, 74, 148, 153–157, 160, 161, 166, 174

Q
Quality improvement (QI), 3–7, 21–27, 37–48, 52, 80, 83–88, 91–99, 104, 106, 112, 113, 130, 132, 187–193, 238, 265–298, 349, 350
Quality improvement resources and journals, 167–168
Quality Interagency Coordination Task Force (QuiC), 12
Qualtrics™, 354, 359
Quasi-experimental studies, 333
Questionnaires and surveys, 25

R
RACI chart. *See* Responsible, accountable, consulted, informed (RACI) chart
Randomized controlled trial (RCT), 333
Red rules, 229
RefWorks, 162
Relationship diagram, 237–238
Residency program director, 41–48
Residents, 10, 37–39
Responsible, accountable, consulted, informed (RACI) chart, 289–290
R for statistics, 364–388
Risk ratio (RR), 334
Root cause analysis, 6, 78, 251, 276, 291
R statistical software, 61, 64
RStudio program, 364, 365
Run chart, 61, 244, 245, 274

S
Safety, 5
Safety assurance (SA), 18
Safety management system (SMS), 17–18
Safety policy, 18
Safety promotion, 18
Safety risk management (SRM), 17–20
SBAR communication tool. *See* Situation, Background Assessment, Recommendation (SBAR) communication tool
Scatter diagram, 243–245
Scope statement, 209
SEIPS model. *See* Systems Engineering Initiative for Patient Safety (SEIPS) model
Sentinel event, 6
SIPOC diagram, 213–215, 278, 280, 310–311
Situational awareness, 228–229

Situation, Background Assessment, Recommendation (SBAR) communication tool, 221–222
  acute care therapy, 118–119
  early-in-day discharge, 92–93
  global immunization core measure, 101–104
  patient discharge communication, 70–71
  patients mobility, 57–59, 65–66
  smoking cessation in pregnancy, 83–86
  stat medication process, 134–136
Six Sigma methodology, 268–271, 318, 386–388
SLP. *See* Speech-language pathologists (SLP)
SMART. *See* Specific, measurable, achievable, relevant, and time bound (SMART)
Smoking cessation in pregnancy, 83–85
SMS. *See* Safety management system (SMS)
Spaghetti diagram, 284, 285
Spearman correlation coefficient, 382–383
Specific, measurable, achievable, relevant, and time bound (SMART), 67
Speech-language pathologists (SLP), 118
SPIKES method, 228
SRM. *See* Safety risk management (SRM)
Stakeholder analysis, 285–286
Stata, 30
Stat medication process, 134–143
Stratification chart, 244, 245
Survey methodology, 353–360
SurveyMonkey™, 354, 359
Swim lane diagram, 279, 282
Systems approach to healthcare, 6
Systems-based model, 47
Systems Engineering Initiative for Patient Safety (SEIPS) model, 22–23

T
Takt Time, 311
Task analysis, 26
Teach-back method, 227
Team assistance, 230
Team-based model, 47
Team building, 255–256
Team creativity, 260–261
Team culture, 287–288
Team huddle, 223
Team management, 255–263
Team Strategies to Enhance Performance and Patient Safety (TeamSTEPPS), 262–263
Teamwork, 45–46
Time and motion studies, 26
Total quality management (TQM), 4
Translating evidence into practice (TRIP) model, 112
Transparency, 5
Tree diagram, 251, 252
T tests, 368–369
Tuckman's stages of group development, 256
Two-challenge rule, 230

U
Unit-based model, 47
URAC, 14

Usability evaluation, 26

V
Value added (VA) map, 309
Value stream map (VSM), 74, 75, 134, 135, 279, 283, 308
Venous thromboembolism (VTE), 336–339
Voice of the Customer (VOC), 73–74, 310

W
Waste Walk, 314, 315
Wilcoxon Rank Sum test, 369, 373
Wow factor, 52, 102
Writing and publishing resources, 167

MIX
Papier aus verantwortungsvollen Quellen
Paper from responsible sources
FSC® C105338
FSC
www.fsc.org

If you have any concerns about our products,
you can contact us on
ProductSafety@springernature.com

In case Publisher is established outside the EU,
the EU authorized representative is:
Springer Nature Customer Service Center GmbH
Europaplatz 3, 69115 Heidelberg, Germany

Printed by Libri Plureos GmbH
in Hamburg, Germany